Navigating the Inequitable U.S. Healthcare System

Navigating the Inequitable U.S. Healthcare System: In Search of Critical Care

Kellina Craig-Henderson

ANTHEM PRESS

Anthem Press
An imprint of Wimbledon Publishing Company
www.anthempress.com

This edition first published in UK and USA 2024
by ANTHEM PRESS
75–76 Blackfriars Road, London SE1 8HA, UK
or PO Box 9779, London SW19 7ZG, UK
and
244 Madison Ave #116, New York, NY 10016, USA

British Library Cataloguing-in-Publication Data
A catalogue record for this book is available from the British Library.

Library of Congress Cataloging-in-Publication Data: 2023952171
A catalog record for this book has been requested.

ISBN-13: 978-1-83998-767-0 (Hbk)
ISBN-10: 1-83998-767-7 (Hbk)

This title is also available as an e-book.

CONTENTS

FOREWORD

In 20 years of marriage, I only remember 4–5 arguments among us. One of the last was her treatment strategy, but it was her body and I eventually understood her rationale later (wanting to get back to normal). Kellina was an elegant, stunningly beautiful, brilliant woman who was extremely humble, yet very intense. She wanted the most out of each minute life had to offer. She was Lois, I was the Clark Kent persona; she was an awesome wife and mother, whom I deeply miss.

To understand how Kellina helped others is simply to contact the National Science Foundation or Google, "NSF mourns Kellina." She had a profound impact on so many people. She encouraged me to publish, to pass on my cybersecurity knowledge to others in order to help develop others and to make strives for cybersecurity best practices. My first publication was "Security Architecture and Models" chapter within Krause, M., & Tipton, H., 2003, *Information Security Management Handbook*, 5th Ed. This was a collaboration with Kellina. She was a social psychologist, and I asked her to write a section on social engineering for cybersecurity practitioners, not her fellow academics or students. I read her social engineering piece and handed it back to her. Kellina thought something was wrong by the expression on my face I suppose. I stated it was an outstanding technical writing on the subject and I had nothing further to add. At the time, Kevin Mitnick was the sought-after thought leader on social engineering. Kellina addressed the subject from the academic side yet in layman terms for cybersecurity practitioners.

I wrote several other publications afterward with her encouragement (all edited by her). She would invite me to National Science Foundation's (NSF) computer science open discussions or public presentations. She told me, for example, research states not to allow a toddler to watch TV before the age of two. That aggression of computer games on developing adolescence minds is harmful. She made me a better father. I can honestly state, Kellina is probably a cofounder on the science, technology, engineering and mathematics (STEM) to what it is today and within the federal government. Her other signature task was broadening the participation of minorities in STEM.

Kellina was a recognized hate crime (justice department expert witness) and an aggression expert, who was well published as a social psychologist and researcher at tier 1 facilities. Afterward, she became Assistant Director for the Social Behavioral and Economic Sciences division at NSF. She was the perfect person to write on the inequality of U.S. healthcare as a social psychologist and from her personal experiences as a minority. She had her sorority sister (medical doctor) and best friend assist her with writing this book. I find it ironic and tragic, for Representative Steven Scalise it was all hands on deck, yet for my beloved wife, it was one misdiagnosis after another, until the late stages of the disease when the treatments finally began.

My involvement was as caretaker, like her father. We thought had more time, but she did not tell me she was actively dying, I later learned. This book was a bucket list action. She explained to me that it was very difficult to write emotionally. I had naively thought she was mentioning what she had gone through. I later came to understand why as I mentioned previously. I kept loving and encouraging Kellina as it was important for her to get this published. She spent inordinate energy to get it to the publisher around August of 2022. Subsequently, she was literally in an out-of-hospitals weeks at a time.I would share *USA Today* or other related articles I would read from my periodical readings. I took up the bulk of the home chores except for cooking dinner, which I outsourced to Door Dash.

I know my wife—she saw a problem, wanted to highlight an issue, and change things on this subject. The publisher contacted me after she passed and I asked a couple of times to get this book published. I am forever grateful. I provided a list of reviewers and performed the final edit while finalizing her estate, raising a son as a single parent, and attended four additional painful funerals after losing her. This publication was very important to her, I loved her dearly, I didn't want to disappoint the love of my life.

Foster

Chapter 1

THE CRISIS OF DIAGNOSIS

Recently, I was diagnosed with a life-threatening rare disease. My efforts to obtain treatment and medical care, though not as difficult as my now daily struggle to survive, reflect the inherent challenges of navigating the U.S. healthcare system and more pointedly so as a woman of color who happens to be an African American. If my life did not depend on obtaining effective treatment, all of these experiences together might have merely proven to be an inconvenience, something I might have complained about as much as I would have complained about the ill-mannered driver who cut me off while driving the other day. And, if it were just a matter of turning to any one of the powerful online search engines that exist to find effective treatment, my ongoing experience would merely resemble an ambitious trek down a mildly interesting path. This was not the case.

Early on, I decided to document and interrogate my observations and experiences about this process in a somewhat happenstance fashion. That is to say that the idea for an ethnography recounting those experiences came later. Prior to this crisis, I could not have imagined knowing about the steps involved in being diagnosed with a life-threatening illness, followed by the desperate searching for treatment and care, and ultimately obtaining life-prolonging treatment.

From the beginning, I kept a small journal in which I recorded this process, highlighting the various situations in which I found myself. I did so because of the challenge I faced in remembering what any one of the doctors and specialists to whom I turned told me. It was all very overwhelming, and the only way I could process the information (sometimes contradictory) that I received was to dutifully record it for later and sometimes multiple reviews. My first entry and each one thereafter included not only what I was told but also my observations about the exchange and my reactions to the doctor. This journal and the notes recorded serve as a basis for this text.

There is a long-standing historical tradition within the realm of qualitative research for this approach to gathering information.

Known as *participant observation*,[1] this approach was most popular at the turn of the twentieth century as the research method of choice for a variety of social scientists, including sociologists and anthropologists.[2] Today, it is often used to uncover elicit or unknown behaviors, lifestyles, and perspectives within settings that most people know little about.[3]

As with any qualitative research project, my analysis is not immune to the risks of subjectivity. As a patient and a recipient of medical treatment and care, I was a complete insider and unable to completely detach from the context of critical care—that is, the research setting.[4] There is also the matter of this being entirely too personal to generalize to any larger group of people. Those qualms aside, what little evidence I can provide represents one snapshot of the healthcare system for critical care.

Perhaps a more apt characterization of what I have attempted to describe here is reminiscent of French sociologist Wacquant's (2006) *observant participation*. In writing of his immersion into the world of amateur and professional boxing engaged in all phases of the pugilist's strenuous training, Wacquant wrote as both boxer and sociologist to provide a compelling picture of the boxing life for poor Black men in Chicago's south side.[5] Another researcher, borrowing from renowned sociologist Ervin Goffman,[6] has also emphasized the value of "going backstage" to gather information as a researcher who is fully immersed in the research setting.[7] Yet, another researcher examining the experience of illicit and illegal street-based drug injection suggests that observant participation contributes toward an enhanced understanding of social problems that surpasses that gained from alternative, less engaged research methods.[8] In the tradition of an observing participant, I provide

1 Bryman, Alan. (2016). *Social Research Methods*. Oxford University Press.

2 As examples of this approach, see work by B. Malinowski, as well as that of F. Boas (1924).

3 As a contemporary example, see Khan, S. R. (2014). *Privilege: The Making of an Adolescent Elite at St Paul's School*. Princeton, NJ: Princeton University Press.

4 Monti, Daniel J. (1992). On the Risks and Rewards of "Going Native". *Qualitative Sociology* 15 (3): 325–332. https://doi.org/10.1007/BF00990332.

5 Wacquant, L. (2006). *Body & Soul*. Notebooks of an Apprentice Boxer. Oxford University Press.

6 Goffman, Ervin. (1967). *Interaction Ritual: Essays on Face-to-Face Behaviour*. New York: Pantheon Books.

7 Wilkinson, C. A. (2017). Going "backstage": Observant Participation in Research with Young People. Children's Geographies 15 (5): 614–620.

8 Parkin, S. (2016). Observant Participation with People Who Inject Drugs in Street-Based Settings: Reflections on a Method used During Applied Ethnographic Research. *Journal Addiction Research & Theory* 25 (1): 39–47.

this analysis of the process of obtaining life-saving critical healthcare as an African American patient and a researcher.

I have chronicled my experiences in seeking and obtaining care, and draw from the principles of qualitative research to make inferences and provide insights about the way that the healthcare system works from the perspective of a critically ill patient.[9] This is an epistemological approach that hinges on (1) the value of the subject matter—systemic barriers to healthcare have been problematized as a result of the COVID-19 pandemic; (2) the clarity of the research inquiry—what is the process by which critical care is obtained; and (3) the behavior and involvement of the researcher—in this case, me. What is most clear from my effort is that there are unintended obstacles (beyond the usual suspects) to obtaining healthcare that have very little to do with my insurance or my ability to pay for my care. Instead, my ability to obtain treatment and care was determined in large part by a constellation of implicit cognitive associations, historic inequities, and systemic and institutional bias. The latter factors, including systemic and institutional bias as well as historic inequities, are embedded within the structure of the healthcare insurance industry.

Nearly two decades ago, the Institute of Medicine (IOM) (2002) issued its report *Unequal Treatment: Confronting Racial and Ethnic Disparities in Healthcare.*[10] What that report made public and surprised many is now readily acknowledged by most today—that racial and ethnic minorities receive lower quality healthcare than White Americans even when they have comparable insurance and their ability to pay is the same. Fast forward 18 years, and in 2020, the COVID-19 pandemic has highlighted the pervasiveness of health inequities as well as the problem of disparate access to healthcare. Those who may have initially questioned the veracity of the 2002 report's findings have even less reason to doubt them given the widespread evidence in local and national contexts of the virus' disproportionate impacts on race and ethnic minorities and the differential value of life for White and people of color as evidenced in the quality of care and treatment received.

9 Alasuutari, Pertti. (2010). The Rise and Relevance of Qualitative Research. *International Journal of Social Research Methodology* 13 (2): 139–155. https://doi.org/10.1080/13645570902966056. S2CID 143736805.

10 IOM report. Unequal Treatment: Confronting Racial and Ethnic Disparities in Health Care (2003). https://nap.nationalacademies.org/login.php?record_id=12875&page=https%3A%2F%2Fnap.nationalacademies.org%2Fdownload%2F12875; IOM. (2002). Unequal Treatment: What Health Care System Administrators Need to Know about Racial and Ethnic Disparities in Healthcare. https://nap.nationalacademies.org/resource/10260/disparities_admin.pdf.

In the intervening years, a number of important books addressing academic and lay audiences exploring the thesis that access to medical care, the health system, quality of life and life expectancies continue to be causally related to such things as race, ethnicity and socioeconomic status have been published with varying acclaim. Foremost among them, Matthew's (2015) *Just Medicine*[11] calls for a "Culture of Health" focused on eradicating inequity in healthcare and presents compelling evidence for the impact of implicit bias and prejudice in healthcare. Its author proposes a series of legal reforms based on scientific research findings about how people behave that, when viewed collectively, have the potential to alter the landscape of healthcare delivery and shift the social norm that has permitted, and even sanctioned, health inequity for so long.

There are several other authors who have contributed to this literature since the 2002 report with equally ambitious texts that, when taken together, describe doctors' thoughts about the meaning of race and its impacts on diagnoses and treatments,[12] identify the way that societal inequalities drive health disparities throughout the world,[13] unveil the history of medical experimentation on African Americans[14] and in the unusual case of a memoir authored by a Black physician, it documents the personal experience as a healthcare provider in a system that does not value Black lives or Black physicians.[15]

A walk through this sobering literature leaves one heavy with the understanding that disparities exist at every step within the healthcare system that make illnesses more dangerous and more deadly for people of color, the poor, and marginalized.[16,17] One need only be a mediocre student of this work to discern that the cost of not being White or economically well off for patients

---

11 Matthew, Dayna Bowen. (2015). *Just Medicine: A Cure for Racial Inequality in American Health Care*, Reprint Edition. New York: New York University Press.

12 Hoberman, John. (2012). *Black and Blue: The Origins and Consequences of Medical Racism.* California: University of California Press.

13 Marmot, Michael. (2015). *The Health Gap: The Challenge of an Unequal World.* New York: Bloomsbury Publishing Co.

14 Washington, Harriet. (2006). *Medical Apartheid: The Dark History of Medical Experimentation on Black Americans from Colonial Times to the Present.* New York: Harlem Moon Publishing.

15 Tweedy, Damon. (2016). *Black Man in a White Coat: A Doctor's Reflections on Race and Medicine.* Paperback—September 6, 2016. New York: Picador Books.

16 Barr, Donald. (2019). *Health Disparities in the United States: Social Class, Race, Ethnicity, and the Social Determinants of Health*, third Edition. Baltimore, MD: Johns Hopkins University Press.

17 Ansell, David. (2019). *The Death Gap: How Inequality Kills.* Chicago, IL: University of Chicago Press.

who are ill is manifested in less engagement with the healthcare industry and that this translates into less care overall. More astute readers of this literature will conclude that any transformation to address these inequities will require a complete overhaul that includes meaningful changes to medical school training, widespread acceptance of punitive measures for discriminatory individual, and institutional-level behaviors, as well as increased access to affordable healthcare for all Americans.

This book and the material presented here start with a fundamental understanding and awareness of these inequities, their impacts and the social and economic costs of a healthcare system that fails to provide equitable care to everyone in need. As a social scientist interested in examining the matter of systemic inequity, I was particularly interested in documenting the impact of racial and ethnic inequities on the quest for critical healthcare in the context of a major healthcare crisis. As a healthcare consumer recently plunged into the marketplace for life-saving healthcare, I systematically explored and documented the process of obtaining care as an African American woman against the backdrop of an emerging global pandemic. This book recounts these experiences by showing specific instances where the ogre of race intruded and influenced my ability to obtain quality care. I was particularly interested in documenting the process by which I was ultimately able to obtain care and the way that I was treated within the medical establishment by its mostly well-intentioned physicians, nurses, and other medical personnel.

In the following pages, across multiple diagnoses, several stages of treatment and medical domains, I report on the process of obtaining life-saving care for a critical illness. Throughout this process, I have documented the efforts required to obtain care and, in doing so, inevitably examined the way that structural inequities and implicit cognitive associations of healthcare practitioners affected my ability to obtain care. There were times when my interaction with medical personnel was helpful and encouraging, and there were times when I was left feeling frustrated, insulted, and hopeless. The challenge in navigating the healthcare industry as a patient in need of life-saving care involves not just the medical staff, including its doctors and nurses, but also the structure of the healthcare system itself, including the medical profession and insurance industry. The latter remains as powerful as any medical specialist in determining the delivery of care.

Not surprisingly, this experience helped me better understand the role of the insurance industry in determining available healthcare. Health insurers are both buyers of medical services (from providers) and sellers of health insurance (to consumers and employers), and as such, they play an important role in determining whether certain treatments or care will be made available to patients seeking care.[18] Throughout this text, I also document the way that the insurance industry influenced my treatment and care.

It is impossible to discuss the role of insurance and the ability to obtain medical care without acknowledging the Patient Protection and Affordable Care Act (PPACA), commonly called Obamacare, which was signed into law in 2010. It represents the most significant overhaul in the U.S. healthcare system since 1965. The PPACA, referred to as the ACA throughout this text, is divided into nine titles and was enacted over different time periods. When taken together, the ACA significantly reduces the number of uninsured Americans and reduces the overall cost of healthcare. Millions of Americans who did not have healthcare insurance coverage before the Act took effect now do.

In my case, I entered the healthcare arena fully stocked with private health insurance through my employer. At no time had I or any family member covered by my plan encountered difficulty in obtaining coverage or been denied approval for a treatment or procedure. I would soon come to discover, upon entering the realm of treatment and life-saving therapeutics, how tenuous the relationship between having insurance and obtaining the most effective care could be.

For specific illnesses like cancer, which kill more Americans each year than anything else, some studies suggest that by expanding insurance coverage, the ACA will ultimately improve cancer-related outcomes.[19] A 2017 study published in the *Journal of the American Medical Association* (*JAMA*) found that the number of patients who were uninsured and recently diagnosed fell by one-third in the ACA's first year.[20] Coverage gains were significant across numerous common cancers, multiple demographic groups, and early-stage and late-stage diseases. These findings suggest that the general increase in coverage seen in the national ACA analyses extends to high-risk populations like those with cancer who are also low income.[21] A recent analysis of the

---

18 Arnold, Daniel & Scheffler, Richard, M. (2017). Market Concentration Insurer Market Power Lowers Prices in Numerous Concentrated Provider Markets. *Health Affairs* 36 (9): 1539–1546. DOI: 10.1377/hlthaff.2017.0552.

19 Sommers, B. D., Gawande, A. A., & Baicker, K. (2017). Health Insurance Coverage and Health—What the Recent Evidence Tells Us. *The New England Journal of Medicine* 377 (6): 586–593.

20 Soni, A., Sabik, L. M., Simin, K., & Sommers, B. D. (2018). Chang in Insurance Coverage Among Cancer Patients Under the Affordable Care Act. *JAMA Oncology* 4 (1): 122–124. https://doi.org/10.1001/jamaoncol.2017.3176.

21 Jemal, A., Lin, C. C., Davidoff, A. J., & Han, X. (2017). Changes in Insurance Coverage and Stage at Diagnosis Among Nonelderly Patients With Cancer After the Affordable Care Act. *Journal of Clinical Oncology* 35: 3906–3915.

Kentucky Cancer Registry examining the relationship between cancer survival rates and health insurance from 1995–98 found that across all cancers included (prostate, breast, colorectal and lung) survival rates for the insured were at least 10 percent greater than for those who were insured.[22] Clearly, insurance matters.

A Fall That Started It All

My journey and experience in obtaining critical healthcare began with a fall. I landed on my back and subsequently experienced excruciating pain. A colleague at work recommended a chiropractor her husband saw and with whom he was pleased. I was desperate for relief, and never having consulted a chiropractor, I was curious to find out whether he could help to alleviate my pain. Like most people who know that chiropractors are not medical doctors, I was somewhat skeptical about the likelihood of relief. Nonetheless, in desperation because of the pain that greeted me daily, I booked the next available appointment.

Since its founding in the late nineteenth century, chiropractic has been the subject of controversy and criticism. Chiropractors were jailed for practicing medicine without a license. For most of its existence, chiropractic has battled with mainstream medicine and struggled with the problem of legitimacy. This is due in part to a lack of empirical evidence supporting the value of spinal manipulation, the main treatment method employed by chiropractors. The evidence that exists is ambivalent in showing that it is effective for any medical condition.[23]

On my first visit to the chiropractor, Dr. Z, who was White and appeared to be in his mid- to late-40s, used x-ray radiography to examine my bone structure. That revealed what appeared to be a small fracture. The doctor was engaging and made direct eye contact, and his conversation frequently turned to current events. I was glad we shared similar political views. The initial observation was followed by a 25-minute session of electric dermal muscle stimulation that would become a regular treatment for me. The doctor explained that, with time, I would notice improvement as a result of this stimulation. He also explained that because of the fracture and the

---

22 McDavid, Kathleen, Tucker, Thomas C., Sloggett, Andrew, & Coleman, Michel P. (2003). Cancer Survival in Kentucky and Health Insurance Coverage. *JAMA Internal Medicine* 163 (18): 213–214.

23 Salehi, Alireza, Hashemi, Neda, Imanieh, Mohammad Hadi, & Saber, Mahboobeh. (2015). Chiropractic: Is it Efficient in Treatment of Diseases? Review of Systematic Reviews. *International Journal of Community Based Nursing & Midwifery* 3 (4): 244–254.

discomfort caused by it, I should plan for about 10 more appointments. That seemed a little odd to me, but the pain in my lower back, now acute after the attention it had just received, quelled any doubts about returning. I booked my next appointment while paying my insurance company's co-payment. I ultimately returned for some six more appointments, all involving a combination of electrical dermal stimulation, vertebral subluxation, and later on even acupuncture.

By the seventh visit, I expressed my frustration and insisted on further imaging, given that I continued to experience pain. With some reluctance, he complied and provided me with a prescription for a CT scan. The results of the CT scan clearly revealed a hairline fracture of the fourth lumbar vertebrae, which the chiropractor explained to me while reviewing the results of the scan with me. It was at this point that he suggested I consult with a spinal pain management company. Because chiropractors emphasize conservative management of the neuromusculoskeletal system without the use of medicines or surgery, given my fracture, he recommended I contact them.

The referral to the spinal pain management center turned out to be an ordinary doctor's office. The surgeon, a middle-aged Middle Eastern man, was kind, though a bit hurried. Though I had waited some 20 minutes for his arrival in the examining room after waiting 15 minutes in the waiting area, it seemed that his goal was to ensure considerably less time in his consultation with me. Ultimately, he gave me a choice between minimal, though invasive, spinal surgery or a referral to a physical therapist. I chose the latter and began to meet weekly with a White woman who, like me, was in her early 50s and was a part of the physical therapy clinic that the surgeon recommended. Sometimes, after leaving my sessions with her, I felt relief, and other times I did not. Three months into our sessions, she suggested I return to the surgeon because of our failure to obtain any long-term success and alleviation of the back pain I continued to experience.

I returned to the surgeon, who then offered me a prescription for a drug that he suggested might bring me relief, but the possible side effects intimidated me. He also recommended that I see a general practitioner (GP) and provided me with a referral for a doctor located in his medical park. Feeling as if I would never get rid of this back pain, I made my way to the GP, who ordered a series of blood tests for me. He was a young Indian man who was very polite, asking what seemed to be an appropriate number and type of questions given my ailment.

The initial results of the blood test were puzzling to the doctor, and he suggested we redo the test. I agreed, but not sensing the severity of the suggestion, I put off a return visit to his office for several months. This would prove to be a life-changing mistake, which I would later come to regret. By the time

I did return to his office nearly four months later, I had begun to experience periodic bouts of swelling in my legs and ankles. This suggested an urgency that I had failed to fully comprehend at the time. Not knowing any better, I attributed the swelling to something minor that was obviously out of sync, and while somewhat uncomfortable, I found that if I elevated my legs for some period of time, the swelling went down. Problem solved.

The GP gently admonished me for not having returned sooner and ordered another round of blood tests. The results of those tests were even more concerning and appeared to confirm his suspicions about there being an underlying problem with my kidneys. He explained that there was something awry, and I needed to see a nephrologist at this point. As he explained this, I pointed out to him that there had also been a darkening of my complexion within the last 6–8 months that seemed more mysterious to me than sinister. He listened but did not seem to consider this observation important.

I understood at this point that somehow the abnormal results of the blood tests were related to my swollen limbs and my change in complexion, but I was clueless about what this all meant. The GP offered no solutions to this mystery. In many ways, my partial ignorance shielded me from the alarm that knowledge about what all this meant would have signaled. That said, I would not have dallied to return for a second round of blood tests if I had even so much as suspected something so serious was amiss. In retrospect, I regret not knowing to take things as seriously as I should have. I also regret that the GP did not follow up with me or impress upon me the potential severity of what he suspected at the outset. I am vexed by this failure on his part to follow up with me.

How and whether physicians aggressively recommend follow-up diagnostic testing has been the subject of concern in debates about the existence of racial and ethnic differences in health outcomes. Several studies exploring health outcomes across critical diseases like cancer and heart disease paint an alarming picture of the continuing problem of racial differences in diagnosis, treatment and follow-up. For example, analysis of data from the National Breast and Cervical Cancer Early Detection Program from July 1, 1991, through September 30, 1995, reveals that racial/ethnic minority women had longer periods from the first abnormal screening to diagnosis and from diagnosis to treatment initiation than White women.[24] There is also evidence of racial differentials in the diagnostic follow-up of abnormal

24 Caplan, L. S., May, D. S., & Richardson, L. C. (2000). Time to Diagnosis and Treatment of Breast Cancer: Results from the National Breast and Cervical Cancer Early Detection Program, 1991–1995. *American Journal of Public Health* 90: 130–134.

screening examinations that might also contribute to a higher disease stage at diagnosis among screened populations.[25] In addition, an analysis of SEER-Medicare data for women diagnosed in 1991 showed that African Americans were significantly less likely than Whites to have a mammogram after their diagnosis and treatment of breast cancer.[26] I cannot help but wonder whether the physician's lack of follow-up with me, given the suspicions he harbored about my initial blood tests, might have been different had I been White.[27]

Because I did not know that the swelling in my legs and feet, the never-ending back pain and the change in my complexion could be connected, and I most certainly didn't think that together they were symptomatic of a life-threatening, incurable, rare disease, I did not think much about any one of these symptoms. As unbelievable as it may seem, and because no one had suggested otherwise, I thought that somehow this was all simply a result of extreme fatigue and eating habits.

I went to the nephrologist because the GP referred me, though I was still not particularly alarmed. The nephrologist, another Indian man who had seen the results of my recent blood tests, initially asked me a series of questions. He took a urine specimen on that first visit and then suggested a fairly invasive test—a kidney biopsy. I agreed to it, believing that this would rule out any number of possibilities.

The biopsy was arranged in short order. There was light anesthesia, a surgical team, and an operating room. My attending nurse was a friendly, upbeat middle-aged White woman who had worked at the hospital for some twenty years. I was grateful for her bedside manner which included concern and reflected her experience and expertise. The procedure took less than an hour. After another hour's mandated recovery, my husband drove me home from the hospital. Except for a slight soreness in my side the following day, I was no worse for the wear and immediately returned to work. The specimen was shipped for analysis to the Mayo Clinic in Minnesota. It would take 3 weeks before I received a diagnosis.

---

25 Chang, S. W., Kerlikowske, K., Napoles-Springer, A., Posner, S. F., Sickles, E. A., & Perez-Stable, E. J. (1996). Racial Differences in Timeliness of Follow-Up after Abnormal Screening Mammography. *Cancer* 78: 1395–1402; and see Carey, P., & Gjerdingen, D. K. (1993). Follow-up of Abnormal Papanicolaou Smears among Women of Different Races. *Journal of Family Practice* 37: 583–587.

26 Schapira, M. M., McAuliffe, T. L., & Nattinger, A. B. (2000). Underutilization of Mammography in Older Breast Cancer Survivors. *Med Care* 38: 281–289.

27 McCarthy, B. D., Yood, M. U., Boohaker, E. A., Ward, R. E., Rebner, M., & Johnson, C. C. (1996). Inadequate Follow-up of Abnormal Mammograms. *American Journal of Preventive Medicine* 12: 282–288.

I continued to do everything that was part of my routine in the time that I awaited a diagnosis. This included waking up at 5:30 a.m. most weekdays to make breakfast for my husband and son, stopping at the gym on the way to work, clocking into the office by 8:45 a.m., and then jumping into any number of evening activities immediately after work. The night of the week determined whether I chauffeured my son to Boy Scouts or swim team practice, attended a women's Bible study, met friends for a happy hour, or had dinner out with my husband. Every Sunday morning, I rose early to prepare my lesson for my Sunday school class. I taught Sunday school in my church to a vibrant group of second graders. I was in no way prepared for the diagnosis I received or for all that was to come.

I had ambled into my fifth decade somewhat unremarkably, with neither a leap nor a rush. One morning, I woke up and found that I was 50. Of course, I was aware of each year of the past decade that had brought me to this point, but the sum of those years hadn't really registered until I turned 50. I neither took my health for granted nor became obsessed with it. My biggest health-related goals were to maintain some muscle tone in my upper body and to be trim enough to fit most size 8 garments. I accomplished this primarily by visiting the gym at least three times during the week, skipping dessert, and eating "lite."

There was some irony to the diagnosis I ultimately received because it was at this point that I had finally achieved my ideal weight, something I'd worked toward for a long time. I now found that I could comfortably fit into any size 8 clothing, and the weight seemed to come off with ease. I was pleased with my size and even more pleased with my dedication to the exercise routine I followed. Only later, when the weight loss far exceeded my size 8 goals, did I realize that this too was a symptom of the disease.

There were more signs. This was the first time people I saw at work commented on my weight loss. In the beginning, it began with compliments. Colleagues I hadn't seen in a couple of weeks who saw me offered compliments, noting how great I looked. Later, still prior to alarm, a few approached me confidentially and asked me, "Hey, you okay? Just noticed how much weight you'd loss […]" I responded truthfully and said, "As far as I knew I was ok."

Some three weeks after the initial biopsy, I returned to the nephrologist. He explained the technicalities of the lab results, describing a disease I had never heard of before. "Is this C-C-CANCER?" I asked fearfully. I struggled to say the word. When I did say it, the loud sound of my heart beating with the accompanying rush of blood I heard behind my temples made it nearly impossible for me to hear my own voice. I didn't hear the doctor's answer. "Is there a cure?" I waited. He eventually spoke, "Well […]" I do not recall him saying much else. "Is this going to kill me?" Nothing, though he looked directly at me and smiled weakly. My eyes welled with tears.

Myeloma-associated AL amyloidosis (am-uh-loi-DO-sis). I had never heard of amyloidosis before, and I was equally dumbfounded about how this had happened to me. This was a rare disease, affecting an estimated 4,000 people per year. Amyloidosis is the quintessential rare disease caused by a buildup of abnormal proteins in the body. With AL amyloidosis, the problem stems from a bone marrow disorder—the bone marrow's plasma cells make abnormal protein antibodies, and if left untreated or mismanaged, it can cause organ failure, making it potentially fatal. The disorder of the bone marrow causes the abnormal proteins, which tend to accumulate and cause problems in other critical places in the body like organs, tissue, and nerves. AL amyloidosis is considered a cancer because it is caused by an abnormal growth of cells.

More than anything else, the doctor was apologetic. He treated me respectfully, even referring to me as "Doctor" throughout our conversation (I have a PhD). He clearly regretted the situation. Like me, he was also reticent; he seemed to call this thing that now plagued me *cancer*. He told me that this was a disease that damaged vital organs, among other things, and that in my case, it had affected my kidneys. There was some urgency to obtaining treatment because the disease might ultimately destroy my kidneys and eventually my heart.

In retrospect, I see that by not characterizing "this disease" as cancer, it afforded me a little bit of psychic leeway from the worst of the possibilities I imagined. I knew that whatever this was *was bad*, but I reasoned (however incorrectly) that if he didn't refer to it as cancer, it wasn't that bad. He was a kind soul, even if he was a less than direct or accurate doctor. He said that he was sorry for me, and he willingly agreed to discuss the results of the biopsy over the phone with my New York-based father. My father would prove to be an incredibly important resource for me during this time, having worked for much of his adult life as a renal nutritionist. He had more questions for the doctor than I knew to ask. I cried quietly as they spoke, my dad on speaker phone, the doctor answering what questions he could in his friendly manner. When they had finished, the doctor agreed to find a referral for me. He admitted to not personally knowing much about the disease but said that he knew someone who knew someone in a practice that he would find out about.

That my diagnosis was associated with multiple myeloma (MM) was not entirely unusual. According to what I later learned about the disease, MM is diagnosed in about 30 percent of cases of AL amyloidosis, and affects some 7 in 100,000 people. Whereas amyloidosis is caused by the protein buildup caused by the malfunctioning cells, MM is caused by the abnormal growth of malfunctioning plasma cells in the bone marrow. Although it was not immediately obvious to me, I later learned that there was some benefit to having this kind of amyloidosis associated with MM.

As far as cancers go, MM is also rare, accounting for less than 2 percent of all cancer diagnoses. Only 48 percent of patients with MM are still alive five years after their diagnosis, but there has been considerable research studying this incurable disease, and several hopeful treatments have emerged in recent years. Nearly double the number with MM now survives beyond 5 years. Some of these treatments have been shown to work well for amyloidosis, which is why AL amyloidosis associated with MM could be viewed somewhat positively. That being said, in those moments with the doctor, hearing this diagnosis of a rare disease for the first time, I felt as if I had just been presented with a death sentence.

Rare diseases, also called health orphans, present a unique challenge to public health and to patients because they have historically received far less attention from the pharmaceutical industry. The passage of the Orphan Drug Act in 1983 and the efforts of the National Commission of Orphan Disease in 1989, along with patient support groups, have helped to raise public awareness and incentivize research aimed at the development of treatment for rare diseases.[28] The results of the commission's hearing with hundreds of stakeholders revealed the many challenges that patients face, from diagnosis to inadequate insurance and coverage of medical expenses to the limited availability of effective treatments.[29] All of this occurs against the backdrop of limited financing for research.

Rare diseases substantially affect life expectancy and quality of life. Patients' access to education, earning and independent living is severely compromised. The disease not only burdens the patient but also their family members. In one questionnaire survey conducted in 17 European countries,[30] 25 percent of the patients reported that it took 5–30 years from the first reported symptoms to a correct diagnosis. Before the final diagnosis, 40 percent of the patients were diagnosed incorrectly, and the remaining received no diagnosis. In a number of cases, inaccurate diagnoses were provided, which led to unnecessary medical interventions including surgery (16 percent), failure to receive the appropriate medical treatment (33 percent), and psychological counseling under the assumption that the symptoms were psychosomatic (10 percent).

28 See the article Why rare diseases are an important medical and social issue.
29 See Reassessing the Orphan Drug Act (1989).
30 Eurordis Care2 study described in CEMARA, an information system for rare diseases (2010).

One-quarter of the respondents reported traveling to another region in order to receive a confirmatory diagnosis, and 2 percent traveled abroad.

Not surprisingly, when facing a life-threatening illness that is a rare disease, finding the right specialist is critical because, if left untreated, the illness is likely to progress and further its debilitating effect on a person's body. In my case, the urgency of time had to do with the impact of this disease on my kidneys. I knew that because the kidneys are critical for survival and because mine were deteriorating, time was of the essence. Well-functioning kidneys operate "behind the scene" so that there is no real conscious awareness of them. It is only when they are not functioning that you become aware of them. In the months leading up to my diagnosis, I had unwittingly become *aware* of my kidneys (e.g., leg swelling, reduced urination). I was acutely aware of the need to find a specialist who could help me soon. I felt very much alone. I needed a doctor, and I needed one that I could trust who knew what they were doing and who would treat me as an individual person worthy of care.

Eventually, within the week, I heard back from the nephrologist, who provided me with a referral to a cancer specialist working within a multi-provider practice in Alexandria, Virginia. Although he did not know him personally, he had heard good things about him. Having started me on this journey by providing me with this diagnosis, the nephrologist referred me to a large, profitable cancer specialists group, and that would be the end of our interaction. This would be my last time speaking with him.

The nephrologist never followed up with me. He did not inquire about my ability to obtain treatment, my condition, my or care. Apart from any personal feelings of reproach I may have entertained, I saw his failure to follow-up as symptomatic of an even greater professional inadequacy. Follow-up is broad and can be represented by any number of behaviors, including watching for complications after a diagnosis is made and a treatment started, monitoring for future recurrences, revising the diagnosis as the condition evolves, or just following up with a patient to inquire about the referral provided. In an interesting commentary describing the value of follow-up and feedback for diagnosis, Schiff highlights the importance of doctors' follow-up behavior.[31]

Neither the general practitioner nor the nephrologist followed up with me. Had the former done so, it is possible that the ultimate impact of the disease upon my kidneys might have been reduced, thereby reducing the overall impacts of the disease. While there is no direct evidence of malfeasance on the part of either doctor involved, it is impossible not to acknowledge the way

31 Schiff, G. D. (2008). Minimizing Diagnostic Error: The Importance of Follow-up and Feedback. *The American Journal of Medicine* 121 (5): S38–S42.

that their respective hands-off approaches to the delivery of healthcare contributed to a less promising outcome for me. As the mystery of the blood tests, leg swelling and complexion changes unfolded, it became clear that the entire sequence of events might have been altered had the GP been more engaged with me. Furthermore, it is also the case that some of the anxiety and uncertainty I faced following the results of the biopsy could have been assuaged with greater engagement by the nephrologist.

Indeed, to fully understand the complexity of the disease, one must see how the delay in follow-up early on, coupled with the failure to consider the implications of a spinal fracture in an otherwise healthy, vibrant person, compounded the prognosis. A warning bell should have alarmed me upon my initial presentation with a spinal fracture, given the absence of any previous bone breaks or fractures. MM damages the bone marrow, resulting in severe bone pain as well as weakness of the bones. The pain I repeatedly complained about to the chiropractor, the surgeon and the physical therapist was symptomatic of much more than a slight fracture of the fourth lumbar. Had anyone thought to consider this, I would not have wasted the nine months collectively spent in physical therapy, unnecessary chiropractic visits and nonproductive consultations. In the end, the physical therapist is to be credited with recommending a return to the surgeon. She was both savvy and compassionate enough to (1) recognize that something else was wrong that physical exercise was not likely to heal, and (2) forgo the additional monies she stood to gain by continuing to see me despite a failure to actually help me.

Hindsight is 20/20

Hindsight is 20/20, of course, and looking back at the steps that brought me to my diagnosis, I can see that there were two barriers that worked in concert against earlier detection. The first was my own failure to connect the proverbial dots. Whether this can be attributed to sheer ignorance or overly optimistic thinking, I gave short shrift to the GP's original suggestion to return to his office for a second round of blood tests. Although I ultimately did so, it was not until nearly 4 months had passed.

The second barrier is represented by the failure of the healthcare professionals to act more aggressively and more conscientiously in their interactions with me. From the chiropractor to the GP to the nephrologist and to the surgeon, there existed a failure to communicate adequately with me and a failure to consider fully what was best for me.

While I have chosen to point out the various ways that the process of diagnosis fell short and the unique ways that my status as an African American woman likely influenced those shortcomings, this kind of disconnect between patient preferences and physicians' practices has been noted more generally in the literature. In a study of Australian cancer patients, researchers investigated patient preferences for communication practices.[32] They sought to examine whether any disparities between these physician guidelines, patient preferences, and patient recollections existed. The most notable disparities between guidelines and the reported experiences of patients relate to perceived delays in receiving the diagnosis and having adequate opportunity to ask their clinician questions. Clearly, I am not alone in experiencing this kind of barrier to treatment.

32 See the article: Hearing the Bad News of a Cancer Diagnosis: The Australian Melanoma Patient's Perspective (2001).

Chapter 2

BLACK WOMEN'S HEALTHCARE

The preceding chapter referred to the Institute of Medicine's (IOM) 2002 groundbreaking report that documented poorer well-being and health outcomes for African Americans and other ethnic and racial minorities relative to Whites.

The IOM report[1] noted that African Americans are sicker and have shorter life spans, and this is not simply a result of income or access to insurance. Instead, what the report made painfully clear was that "racial and ethnic minorities receive lower-quality health care than white people—even when insurance status, income, age, and severity of conditions are comparable." According to the IOM report, Black people within the United States were less likely than White people to be given appropriate cardiac care, to receive kidney dialysis or transplants, and to receive the best treatments for stroke, cancer, or AIDS. According to the report, "Some people in the United States were more likely to die from cancer, heart disease, and diabetes simply because of their race or ethnicity, not just because they lack access to health care."

Within the United States, structural inequities that exist result from the various systems of oppression that have ensured the continued maintenance of the status quo.[2] The status quo in the United States is one that has historically privileged Whites relative to all others, men relative to women, the rich relative to the poor and working class, and the able-bodied relative to

---

1 IOM report. Unequal Treatment: Confronting Racial and Ethnic Disparities in Health Care. (2003). https://nap.nationalacademies.org/login.php?record_id=12875&page=https%3A%2F%2Fnap.nationalacademies.org%2Fdownload%2F12875; IOM. (2002). Unequal Treatment: What Health Care System Administrators Need to Know about Racial and Ethnic Disparities in Healthcare. https://nap.nationalacademies.org/resource/10260/disparities_admin.pdf.

2 See the Lancet series: Structural racism and health inequities in the USA: evidence and interventions. Bailey, Z., Krieger, N., Agénor, M., Graves, J., Linos, N., & Bassett, M. T. (2017). https://doi.org/10.1016/S0140-6736(17)30569-X.

the disabled.[3,4] Although the definition of who is considered White has varied over the centuries of America's existence,[5] far less mutable has been the belief in White superiority and the right to White privilege. Current discourse about White privilege has focused on inequity in healthcare, racism and justice, education, employment, intimate partner violence, and wealth.[6]

Most people today who are inclined to think about these issues accept this as a reality. In many ways, it has come to be viewed as a part of the "tax" of being a person of color and, in particular, a Black person in the United States. Much like the "tax" that is a part of law enforcement traffic stops for Black drivers, the healthcare and well-being tax is another given. This is not to say that those affected most are complacent or resigned to this state of affairs. To the contrary, among those most aware, there are expressions of anger and outpourings of grief.[7] Indeed, in the wake of the murder of George Floyd, more than a thousand protests took place over the course of two weeks across America.[8] George Floyd epitomized the countless number of Black and Brown victims who lost their lives at the hands of law enforcement.

---

3 Feagin, J. R., & Vera, H. (2018). Future Challenges: The Sociology of Racial and Ethnic Relations, pp. 429–434. Part of the Handbooks of Sociology and Social Research book series (HSSR).

4 Black, L., & Stone, D. (2011). Expanding the Definition of Privilege: The Concept of Social Privilege. *Journal of Multicultural Counseling and Development.* https://doi.org/10.1002/j.2161-1912.2005.tb00020.x.

5 Hacker, A. (2003). *Two Nations: Black and White, Separate, Hostile, Unequal.* New York: Scribner.

6 Rothenberg, Paula S. (Ed.). (2008). *White Privilege*; Branscombe, N. R., Schmitt, M. T., & Schiffhauer, K. (2006). Racial Attitudes in Response to Thoughts of White Privilege. *European Journal of Social Psycho logy* 37: 203–215; Donnelly, D., Cook, K. J., Ausdale, D., & Foley, L. (2005). White Privilege, Color Blindness, and Services to Battered Women; Blanchett, W. J. (2006). Disproportionate Representation of African American Students in Special Education: Acknowledging the Role of White Privilege and Racism; Stone, J. (2002). Race and Healthcare Disparities: Overcoming Vulnerability 23: 499–518.

7 See, for example, https://www.washingtonpost.com/politics/poll-black-americans-outraged-by-george-floyds-death-but-optimistic-about-change-after-nationwide-protests/2020/06/24/1daad46a-b49e-11ea-a510-55bf26485c93_story.html. And: https://www.npr.org/2021/04/13/986678488/grief-outrage-follow-another-police-killing-of-a-black-man.

8 See Sugrue, T. 2020 is not 1968: To understand today's protests, you must look further back. Floyd was one of approximately 1,100 people killed annually by police use of force in the United States in recent years, according to data compiled by Fatal Encounters, a nonprofit that tracks police-involved deaths since 2000. A disproportionate number of the people killed, like Floyd, are African American.

If there has been any silver lining associated with the crisis of the COVID-19 pandemic in America, it has been the unveiling of the disparities that have resulted in greater vulnerability and death for people of color from COVID-related symptoms. As stories unfold detailing the manner in which life-saving care differs or has been unavailable for many in the United States, so too has acknowledgment and acceptance of the belief in healthcare racial inequities expanded.

As local and national news coverage increasingly included reference to the problem of health inequities within the United States, public health officials and some policymakers offered recommendations, directed blame, and collectively expressed outrage over what had existed long before the pandemic but had only become visible during the pandemic.[9] The pandemic has removed the veil that shrouded the many health-related inequities between Whites and ethnic and racial minorities.

Although the disparities between Whites and people of color in the United States were never invisible, it has been possible for most Americans to ignore them. In these cases, the disparities existed just out of direct sight, somewhere beneath the surface of the things that mattered. For those with access to resources and their accompanying privileges, it has historically been convenient to shield one's vision from the unpleasantness of the disenfranchised, the impoverished, and the needy. It is as simple as driving an alternate route to avoid the homeless population or switching the television channel to avoid a documentary detailing suffering someplace in the world. The COVID-19 pandemic lifted whatever blinders existed and brought the reality of inequities into focus. Indeed, it has taken the danger and toll of a viral pandemic to make it clear for all to see the fragility of well-being and survival in many minority communities.

As of today, nearly one million Americans have lost their lives to the deadly virus, with thousands more deaths underreported.[10] While Whites make up the greatest number of victims who die from COVID-19, African Americans

9 American Heart Association. (May 2020). *COVID-19 has Unmasked Significant Health Disparities in the U.S.* https://www.sciencedaily.com/releases/2020/05/200504171856.htm. See too https://www.cnn.com/2021/05/20/health/racial-disparities-covid-19-vaccinations/index.html *Stark Racial Disparities Persist in Vaccinations, State-Level CDC Data Shows.* Retrieved May 28, 2021; https://www.cnn.com/2021/03/10/health/disparities-covid-19-cases-cdc-study/index.html; *Racial Disparities in Covid-19 Case Rates among Young People Were Prevalent Early in the Pandemic, CDC Study Says.* Retrieved May 28, 2021.

10 Centers for Disease Control and Prevention. See https://covid.cdc.gov/covid-data-tracker/.

and Hispanics have a higher risk of infection and die at a greater rate, suggesting the influence of non-disease variables.[11] These variables likely predate the pandemic and are associated with specific ways that minorities interact with the medical system and its healthcare professionals, as well as the economic and other institutional barriers that have ultimately limited mobility and access to effective care. Added to these factors, African Americans and Hispanics are more likely to work in jobs that do not accommodate remote work. For African Americans, whose collective experience includes the legacy of slavery followed by hundreds of years of generational existence in an infrastructure of oppression, it is also the prevalence of co-morbidities like diabetes, hypertension, obesity, and coronary heart disease that increases the risk for COVID-19 and mortality.[12]

African American Women

Many of those inequities are particularly evident in the diagnosis, treatment, and care of Black women.[13] A review of various healthcare concerns reveals a troubling pattern. At every stage of treatment and care, Black women suffer. Consider that Black women are underrepresented in clinical trials that include consent, yet they are overrepresented in studies that do not.[14] FDA data shows that in trials for 24 of the 31 cancer drugs approved since 2015, fewer than 5 percent of participants were Black. It is impossible to test the safety and effectiveness of new drugs for all patients without an adequate representative sample of participants. In contrast, Black participants are disproportionately overrepresented in studies that lack consent or are otherwise unethical.[15]

Consider the 2017 movie *The Immortal Life of Henrietta Lacks,* which revealed the little-known story of the Black woman Henrietta Lacks and her unique

11 Golestaneha, l., Neugartena, J., Fishera, M., Billet, H., Gil, M. R., Johns, T., Yunesa, M., Mokrzyckia, M., Cocoa, M., Norris, K., Perez, H., Scott, S., Kim, R., & Belling, F. (2020). The Association of Race and COVID-19 Mortality. *EClinicalMedicine* 25. https://doi.org/10.1016/j.eclinm.2020.100455.

12 Selden, T. M., & Berdahl, T. (2020). COVID-19 and Racial/Ethnic Disparities in Health Risk, Employment, and Household Composition. *Health Affairs* 39: 8. https://doi.org/10.1377/hlthaff.2020.00897.

13 Williams, D. R. (2008). Racial/Ethnic Variations in Women's Health: The Social Embeddedness of Health. *American Journal of Public Health* 98 (Suppl 1): S38–S47. https://doi.org/10.2105/ajph.98.supplement_1.s38.

14 Consider the epitome of this neglect in the unethical mining and harvesting of Henrietta Lacks' cells.

15 "The Disparities in Healthcare for Black Women."

cell line. The movie was adapted from the similarly titled 2015 meticulously researched text and details the life story of a poor Southern tobacco farmer whose short-lived battle with cervical cancer resulted in the unknowing harvesting and eventual commercialization of her cells.[16] Those cells were cultured and subsequently used to facilitate groundbreaking research in cancer, AIDS, Parkinson's disease, gene mapping, salmonella, hereditary genetic disorders, tuberculosis, and many other medical discoveries.[17]

Unfortunately, many other examples exist of the medical profession's cruelty and wanton disregard for African American women's bodies. Consider the infamous "Mississippi appendectomies" that systematically sterilized poor Black women without their knowledge or consent under the guise of appendectomies during the early twentieth century. Rather than removing their appendixes, doctors performed hysterectomies to prevent poor Black women from reproducing and to provide practical experience for inexperienced doctors.

There are several articles and books that have been published that shed light on the pervasiveness of U.S. policies that forced sterilization on Black women and other women of color.[18] As part of a wider eugenics strategy, Southern states like Mississippi, North Carolina and Virginia employed sterilization as a means of controlling the African American populations.[19]

Perhaps more well-known are the continuing differences in maternal mortality between Black and White women, with Black women experiencing higher rates of maternal mortality and injury regardless of income or education level.[20] Why do Black women die from pregnancy-related complications at 3–4 times higher rates than White women do?[21] And why are they also

16 Skloot, R. (2015). *The Immortal Life of Henrietta Lacks.* New York: Crown Publishing Group.

17 Summerside, M. (2017). From Henrietta to HeLa: A History of Racism and Reality of Distrust in the American Medical System.

18 Stern, A. M. (2005). Sterilized in the Name of Public Health. Race, Immigration, and Reproductive Control in Modern California. Also, Ruteki, G. (2010). Forced Sterilization of Native Americans: Late Twentieth Century Physician Cooperation with National Eugenic Policies.

19 See Boggs, B., & Stone, O. (2013). For the Public Good: The Shameful History of Forced Sterilization in the U.S.

20 Centers for Disease Control and Prevention. (1995). Difference in Maternal Mortality among Black and White Women, United States (1990); Fang, J., Madhavan, S., & Alderman, M. H. (2000). Maternal Mortality in New York City: Excess Mortality of Black Women.

21 Oparah, J. C., & Bonaparte, A. D. (2015). Birthing Justice: Black Women, Pregnancy and Childbirth.

more likely to suffer from a severe disability resulting from childbirth than White women?[22] According to one researcher who has studied the birth stories of African American women, obstetric racism—a threat to positive birth outcomes—is to blame.[23] It best captures the particularities of Black women's reproductive care during the pre- and post-natal period.

There are other areas where disparities are evident. Black women experience disparities in infertility rates, stigmatization and access to fertility care. Infertility affects at least 12 percent of women of childbearing age, and studies suggest this number doubles for Black women in the United States. However, while more than 20 percent of Black women may experience infertility, only 8 percent of them seek medical help to get pregnant, compared to 15 percent of White women.[24]

Consider health maladies that disproportionately impact Black women, such as uterine fibroids. Research on this condition receives very little government funding, and this underscores the reality that Black women's healthcare is not prioritized. Most estimates suggest that nearly a quarter of Black women between the ages of 18 and 30 have fibroids—compared with 7 percent of White women. By age 35, that number increases to 60 percent. Unfortunately, NIH annual funding for the condition is $17 million—compared to $86 million for cystic fibrosis, which happens to impact significantly fewer people each year (though the great majority of those impacted are White).

Precision medicine also appears to be perpetuating disparities. Precision medicine is a relatively recent name for treating disease and providing treatment according to the individual variability in genes, environment, and lifestyle for each person. Consider that genomic research has become a key biomedical resource, and yet genomic datasets contain very few Black women who remain significantly underrepresented in genomic data repositories and related analyses. Indeed, nearly 80 percent of all individuals included in genomic studies are of European descent. While this may be a decrease from 20 years ago (when it was as high as 96 percent), this change is mostly driven by a higher number of studies being done in Asia on populations of Asian ancestry. The increase in participants of African ancestry has barely shifted in the last two decades.[25]

---

22 The Black Women's Health Imperative. See 2020–2021 Policy Agenda. https://3hqwxl1mqiah5r73r2q7zl1l-wpengine.netdna-ssl.com/wp-content/uploads/2021/01/BWHI_NHPA_2020-21.pdf.

23 Davis, D. A. (2018). *Obstetric Racism: The Racial Politics of Pregnancy, Labor, and Birthing.*

24 Davis, R., & Hilmantel, R. (2018). This Is Why We Chose To Talk About Black Women And Infertility.

25 Popejoy, A. B., & Fullerton, S. M. (2016). Genomics is Failing on Diversity.

When one focuses on rates of funding and federal investment in healthcare, a picture emerges reflecting clear disparities in women's health funding, research, delivery, data collection and care, and most relevant for the present discussion, these differences are magnified for women of color and African Americans in particular. Addressing the well-being, treatment and care of Black women would go miles in lifting healthcare for all women.

My Quest for Healthcare

Although my initial diagnosis predated the pandemic's outbreak in the United States by several months, I began the journey to obtain treatment well aware of the problem of differential access as well as the various ways that historical inequities exert a powerful influence on current healthcare disparities. My apprehension over finding a healthcare provider who operated within a system that would have my best interests at heart, treat me as an individual and be absent the refuse of systemic racism and racial prejudice, which I was loath to encounter but knew to exist, nearly immobilized me. In the days that I waited for the nephrologist's referral, I decided to conduct my own search for a specialist in earnest.

Living in the Washington, D.C., metro region, I turned to the renowned, world-famous Johns Hopkins University (JHU) Cancer Hospital in Baltimore, Maryland.[26] Nearly an hour's drive from my home in northern Virginia, the hospital center is known for its cutting-edge research and life-saving treatments. After an hour spent scouring their website, I found a highly esteemed oncologist whose biography and list of specialties included amyloidosis. I began the process of scheduling an appointment.

My relief at having identified a doctor at Johns Hopkins was to be short-lived, and this proved to be a formidable challenge early on during this trial. I learned that doctors who are listed as available specialists at this world-famous hospital are highly selective about which patients they opt to see. I learned this only after multiple phone calls and having left numerous messages. At one point, I nearly broke down on the phone with a scheduling technician. Like me, she was not having a good day. She made it clear that the doctor with whom I was unsuccessfully trying to schedule an appointment was extremely busy and would let me know if she was interested in making an

26 Hopkins' history of providing care to African Americans is complex. It was one of the few that did so, though it did so under strict segregation and with little regard for patient consent. See the book *The Immortal Life of Henrietta Lacks* for an example of Hopkins' performance and engagement with one African American.

appointment with me. Bottom line: I would hear from her about an appointment *if* the doctor decided to see me.

I hung up the phone in disbelief. Was this really happening? It was hard not to take the doctor's brush-off personally, despite it being conveyed through the technician. I knew that there were huge problems with America's healthcare system, and that millions of people either received none or inferior health care because they didn't have insurance or had to make difficult choices between the cost of insurance and other necessities. But what I did not know was that even with "good" insurance, which I thought that I had, and living in the seat of the nation's capital, the ability to obtain satisfactory health care could be so tenuous.

After having shared news of this exchange with my father, he promptly contacted the patient advocacy office at Johns Hopkins to file a complaint. The very next day, I received a phone call and an apology that included a promise that someone would contact me to schedule an appointment. True to her word, I received a call from the very same scheduling technician I'd spoken with previously. With no acknowledgment of our previous conversation, she proceeded to schedule an appointment for me when the doctor was next available. That appointment was scheduled for some 3 months into the future, despite the urgency of my condition.

Around this time, I heard back from the nephrologist, who referred me to cancer specialists of Northern Virginia. I contacted them that very same day but was soon disappointed to learn that the doctor he recommended would be unavailable for nearly six weeks. When I expressed concern about the wait and the urgency of my condition, the office scheduler suggested I see another doctor in their group, a junior associate. She would be available in two weeks. Feeling desperate, I scheduled an appointment with her. I did so reluctantly because the nephrologist had specifically referred me to the doctor, who had nothing less than a six-week wait. As it was, I would have to wait two full weeks before the junior colleague could see me. Feeling as if I had no other options, I scheduled the appointment.

Two weeks later, my husband accompanied me to the appointment. As we walked into the office, I was taken aback by the crowded waiting area. Almost all, that is, 18 of the 20 seats, were filled. With a few exceptions, most of the patients appeared to be White. We took the remaining seats and waited. Nearly 45 minutes later, and after completing some 20 forms attached to a clipboard, we were ushered into a room where, within minutes, we were joined by Doctor "C."

Dr. C was a youthful-looking Asian woman who appeared to be anywhere from her late 20s to early 30s. She was professional and polite, and she wasted no time on pleasantries. She was neither friendly nor warm. Her first words to me were, asked matter-of-factly with no smile, "So, how much do you know about this disease?" I had the feeling (however misplaced it may have been) that how I answered this would determine which category she put me into and how much value and effort she was likely to expend in treating me.

As our conversation proceeded, I was aware of her implicit assessment of me. I felt the gulf that our perceived differences implied. She was young and Asian, and her role as a doctor dictated her advantage within the power dynamic of the doctor-patient relationship. I was fairly certain that her experiences with someone like me, Black, middle-aged and well-educated were fairly limited. I recalled the absence of other patients of color in the crowded waiting room. Doctor "C" assumed certain things about me, which influenced how and what she communicated to me. In fairness, I also assumed some things about her.

The way that people interact with one another is influenced by the "implicit" and "automatic" mental processes that shape their everyday lives.[27] These mental processes exist just below the surface of what is spoken between people and often (though not always) exist outside of conscious awareness or control. Even though these mental processes may exist outside conscious awareness, they exert a powerful influence on our nonverbal behaviors and communication with others. These mental processes, called implicit biases, have increasingly been used to explain the contemporary brand of hostility and antagonism across a broad spectrum of contexts. For example, current explanations for heightened police violence against African American citizens focus on the problem of implicit biases, as do explanations for observed microaggressions in the workplace and school settings.[28] While critics of this perspective have appropriately argued that the problem of racial prejudice runs deeper and is more sinister than any one person's mental baggage,[29] the existence of implicit bias, particularly within the healthcare setting, remains very real.

Consider the results of one study in which physicians rated their perceptions of patients' intelligence, education, self-control, pleasantness, rationality,

---

27 Devine, P. (2001). Implicit Prejudice and Stereotyping: How Automatic are they? Introduction to the Special Section.

28 Carbado, D., & Rock, P. (2016). What Exposes African Americans to Police Violence; and Brunson, R. K. (2007). "Police don't like black people": African-American Young Men's Accumulated Police Experiences.

29 See, for example: Selmi, M. (2018). The Paradox of Implicit Bias and a Plea for a New Narrative. *Arizona State Law Journal* 50: 193.

independence, and responsibility.[30] They also rated their patients on the basis of their perceptions of patient behavior as well as their feelings of affiliation with them. Results showed that physicians were less likely to have positive perceptions of Black patients across multiple attributes. They rated Black patients as less intelligent, less educated, less compliant, and more at risk. This work demonstrates the power of cultural stereotypes and bias to influence physicians' impressions even before the clinical encounter.

The study of biases and implicit cognitive associations, as they are technically called, has a very rich and robust evidentiary base.[31] Many empirical studies have demonstrated that people hold beliefs about others that are associated with their membership in certain groups and are linked to positive and negative feelings that exist just below their conscious awareness.[32] Those positive and negative feelings shape our thoughts about others and influence the nature of our interactions and anticipated interactions with members of those groups. When the biases associated with a group are negative, the outcome is disparate treatment, discrimination, or neglect.

Implicit biases have been identified across a range of different types of social groups, including racial and ethnic minorities, women and sexual minorities, religious groups, athletes, firefighters, the disabled, the obese, the physically attractive, and more. Because of the way that people process information and make sense of the world, there are many potential biases that are possible. Thus, people tend to form biases about others on the basis of well-known characteristics about which a person has no or very little control (e.g., race, gender, age).

In the context of the healthcare industry, research has found that implicit biases are associated with race, ethnicity, gender, age and weight, among other things.[33] What matters most is the way that these biases may influence

30 Van Ryn, M., & Burke, J. (2000). The Effect of Patient Race and Socioeconomic Status on Physicians' Perceptions of Patients. *Social Science and Medicine* 50: 813–828.

31 Greenwald, Anthony G., & Banaji, Mahzarin R. (1995). Implicit Social Cognition: Attitudes, Self-Esteem, and Stereotypes. *Psychological Review* 102 (1): 4–27; Blair IV, et al. (2011). Unconscious (implicit) Bias and Health Disparities: Where Do We Go from Here? *Permanente Journal* 15 (2): 71–78.

32 There are a number of examples of these, including Aboud, F. E., & Doyle, A.-B. (1996). Parental and Peer Influences on Children's Racial Attitudes; Barden, J., Maddux, W. W., Petty, R. E., & Brewer, M. B. (2004). Contextual Moderation of Racial Bias: The Impact of Social Roles on Controlled and Automatically Activated Attitudes; and Snyder, M., Tanke, E. D., & Berscheid, E. (1977). Social Perception and Interpersonal Behavior: On the Self-Fulfilling Nature of Social Stereotypes.

33 FitzGerald, C., & Hurst, S. (2017). Implicit Bias in Healthcare Professionals: A Systematic Review; Dehon, Erin, Weiss, Nicole, Jones, Jonathan, Faulconer, Whitney,

the quality and treatment of patients to the extent that they either possess features characteristic of or are members of stigmatized groups that are associated with negative implicit biases. When healthcare providers harbor implicit biases, they contribute to the problem of healthcare disparities.[34] Most of the research examining implicit bias in healthcare settings concludes that people of color face disparities in access to healthcare, the quality of care received, and health outcomes.[35]

In her groundbreaking text, *Just Medicine*, Dayna Bowens Matthew highlights the role of implicit racism in reviewing the preponderance of evidence showing that doctors' disparate treatment of minority patients is associated with their biases. In this analysis, implicit racism is a primary contributor to health disparities. The doctors' implicit racism can lead to discrimination in a number of ways—from being less aggressive about encouraging a patient to modify risk behaviors to declining to refer a patient to a specialist and instead recommending a more conservative, less ambitious approach to treatment. Their implicit biases are evident throughout the consultative and decision-making processes. There is also evidence that physicians are more likely to delay consultation and refrain from diagnostic testing early for patients of color. Thus, there are multiple points at which doctors' biases can result in discrimination against minority patients, and ultimately inferior care, whether resulting from consciously held beliefs about the value of a particular minority group or unconsciously held attitudes and beliefs about people of color relative to Whites.

As I sat across from Dr. C, I was painfully aware of this, and I considered the matter of the apparent gulf between the two of us. Biases are more likely to influence interactions and behaviors when people have less familiarity and interact with those from different social groups and those they do not know well. Apart from what she read in my chart indicating my diagnosis and my appearance, she knew very little about me. I knew even less about her.

I realized that a fair amount of time would need to be spent getting past her pre-existing beliefs about me, about African Americans, and about

Hinton, Elizabeth, & Sterling, Sarah. (2017). Academic Emergency Medicine. A Systematic Review of the Impact of Physician Implicit Racial Bias on Clinical Decision Making. https://doi.org/10.1111/acem.13214.

34 Narayan, Mary Curry. (2019). Addressing Implicit Bias in Nursing: A Review. *American Journal of Nursing* 119 (7): 36–43. https://doi.org/10.1097/01.NAJ.0000569340.27659.5a.

35 Hall, William J., Chapman, Mimi V., Lee, Kent M., Merino, Yesenia M., Thomas, Tainayah W., Payne, B. Keith, & Eng, Eugenia. (2015). Implicit Racial/Ethnic Bias Among Health Care Professionals and Its Influence on Health Care Outcomes: A Systematic Review. *American Journal of Public Health*, December.

middle-aged African American women in general. And, because communication is a two-way street, I would also need to suspend any stereotypic beliefs that I had formed about her. It was going to take a considerable amount of time to *warm* things up. Although I made a follow-up appointment before leaving her office at the request of the receptionist, I was pretty certain that as I left there, I would not be returning.

I found the doctor's apparent lack of compassion to be especially troubling. Throughout the questions she asked me and in all the information she presented to me there was an absence of compassion or sympathy. Perhaps she did not see it as her responsibility to express sympathy to her patients. Perhaps her focus on developing a treatment plan overshadowed her ability to offer as much. Whatever accounted for her disposition, I knew that this situation in which she, as the doctor, was describing the prognosis expected for a non-curable, life-threatening disease to me, as the patient now confronting the likelihood of my own mortality, warranted some measure of sympathy. The fact that her words fell flat and lacked any hint of compassion compromised our rapport and ability to connect within the doctor-patient relationship. I was even more anxious following my visit with Dr. C because I did not know where else to turn or whether there were any other options for treatment for me.

This issue of communication between doctors and their patients has been the subject of several empirical studies. In one study, communication between the patient and physician was less effective when the patient was of lower socioeconomic status, as determined by occupation or insurance coverage.[36,37] That study highlighted the way that demographic differences and the doctor-patient perceptions surrounding them can compromise their communication and quality of interaction.

This matters because the quality of communication between the doctor and patient directly impacts the treatment and outcome for the patient.[38] Not surprisingly, better communication is associated with better overall experiences for patients. For example, one study found that knowledge about the quality of doctor-patient communication strongly predicted the quality of

36 See Effects of patients' socioeconomic status and physicians' training and practice on patient-doctor communication.

37 Ong, L. M., de Haes, J. C. J. M., Hoos, A. M., & Lammes, F. B. (1995). Doctor-Patient Communication: A Review of the Literature.

38 Bensing, J. (1991). Doctor-Patient Communication and the Quality of Care.

psychosocial care and patient satisfaction.[39,40] A substantial literature exists detailing the value of communication in the doctor-patient relationship and its association with patient outcomes, satisfaction, and compliance with recommendations for care.[41] And, although I was unaware of this at the time of my consultation with Doctor "C," it is clear that our interaction suffered as a result of communication failure. Whether that in turn resulted from our apparent differences or not, it affected the nature of her communication with me. Like a self-fulfilling prophecy, I responded in turn to her less-than-personable demeanor.

I was acutely aware of Dr. C's lack of warmth and what I perceived to be her failure to see me as someone worthy of her unique consideration. After "quizzing" me on my knowledge of the disease, she dispassionately delivered a likely prognosis and initial plan for treatment that left me feeling even more ill at ease than I had upon arrival. I wondered to what degree our perceived differences influenced her interaction. It is possible that, because of the heightened anxiety and overarching concerns I had about obtaining care, I was being overly sensitive. On the other hand, as an African American woman seeking care, I was sensitive to the potential impact of stereotyping and perceived bias in the initial doctor-patient consultation.

Compounded Challenges

Recent research by the medical anthropologist Tina Sacks reports similar reactions among participants in a study documenting the way that middle-class Black women engage health care providers. Beyond analyzing Black–White health disparities, her book describes the healthcare experiences of a sample of 30 Black middle-class women. Based on in-depth focus groups and individual interviews, she shows that Black women feel that they must prepare themselves mentally, emotionally and physically before they ever enter the doctor's office. They dress carefully, emphasize their prestigious careers and make it clear that they have researched their own situation. All of this enables them to be better able to confront what they anticipate their provider's potentially biased opinions and stereotypes about them will be. According to the author, study participants shared that they had encountered providers

39 Matusitz, J., & Spear, J. (2014). Effective Doctor–Patient Communication: An Updated Examination.

40 Buller, M. K., & Buller, D. B. (1987). Physicians' Communication Style and Patient Satisfaction.

41 Trust and Communication in a Doctor Patient Relationship: A Literature Review. (2018).

who disregarded their concerns about their health or advised unnecessarily invasive procedures that did not match the severity of their health concerns. This study shows the ways that Black women face discrimination throughout the healthcare system—from when they enter a medical office to long after they leave.

For ethnic and racial minorities who experience major illnesses or health crises, there are clearly unique challenges to obtaining quality healthcare. Even with insurance and the ability to pay, they receive a lower quality of care than their White counterparts. This racial difference, akin to a racial tax, is evident at each phase of the process of obtaining care. From initial consultation and diagnosis to referral, treatment and actual follow-up. There are many ways that this happens, and while there remain instances in which intentional decisions lead to inferior treatment and care for minorities, there are many more unintentional decisions that have these outcomes. According to the IOM report, it is the unconscious biases and implicit associations that healthcare providers have about patients that ultimately dictate their behaviors and policies as well as influence the quality of care provided.[42]

The book *Black Man in a White Coat* provides a first-hand account of the way that biases throughout the medical profession affect people's behavior as patients and healthcare providers.[43] Its author, a physician, recounts a range of racial slights and insults experienced on a daily basis as an African American physician working in today's healthcare system. He provides a disturbing account of the insidious nature of racism, whether subtle (as in the case of implicit bias) or direct, as when a patient who is assigned to him openly questions his credibility as a physician because he is Black. The narrative illustrates just how comfortably racism and racial bias continue to exist in settings where Black and Whites interact with one another. From the patients who refused to speak directly to him, to fellow doctors who assumed he was a janitor, the fact of his racial status defined the interactions he had when delivering care to patients and when consulting with colleagues.

Getting to Know You

At the very first consultation between the doctor and the new patient, there is a kind of "getting to know you" stage during which the patient presents themselves to the doctor, who not only takes in what the patient says to them but also spends as much time attending to unspoken "cues" about the patient.

42 IOM report (2002).
43 See the book Black Man in a White Coat (2015) by Damon Tweedy.

It is these unspoken cues that will determine the doctor's overall perception of the patient. Whether they are largely consistent with the stereotype the doctor has about people like the patient or not will, in turn, influence, however unconsciously, the doctor's approach to communicating and interacting with the patient.

There is also the difference in status that heightens the potential interaction challenges in the doctor-patient initial consultation. The doctor enters the interaction with a higher status resulting from their expertise, and when the patient is from a racial minority group and the doctor is not, the existing status difference is enhanced. Of course, given the demographic landscape of the American medical profession today, it is just as likely that a patient who is a minority person will be treated by a doctor who happens to be a first- or second-generation American minority person (e.g., Indian American). Unfortunately, even if the doctor happens to be a person of color, such as an Indian American, because of the ubiquity of racism, this initial consultation also requires a kind of "translation" and "getting to know you" phase that can potentially delay the doctor's most ambitious treatment for the patient.

Because of this state of affairs, recommendations abound from studies whose findings suggest that more diversity among healthcare providers leads to a reduction in the healthcare disparities that currently exist, with people of color receiving inferior and less desirable care than Whites. The implications of this for minority healthcare consumers are sobering. In 2008, roughly 75 percent of the medical school graduates practicing medicine were White. The remaining percentage included Asians (12.8 percent), African Americans (6.3 percent), American Indians/Alaska Natives (0.5 percent) and Hispanics (5.5 percent) in the U.S. physician workforce. By 2016, a census of actively licensed allopathic and osteopathic physicians in the United States revealed that there were 953,695 serving a national population of 323 million people. According to the Federation of State Medical Boards (FSMB), this reflects an increase of 12 percent from 2010 to 2016 in the number of physicians licensed to practice medicine throughout the country. Despite this observed increase, there remain relatively fewer practicing physicians of color. If every minority healthcare consumer wanted a physician who shared their racial status, only a small fraction of them would actually be able to have one.

When doctors see patients who have a similar race status as themselves, there is less time needed in the "getting to know you" phase. Just as doctors with a dissimilar race background make assumptions and form stereotypes about patients, so too do those with similar race status. The difference in stereotypes is that they are less likely to be negative and all-encompassing. It makes sense then that doctors with a similar race status as their patients will be more likely to hear, interpret and understand their patients' complaints or concerns. Not surprisingly, research in clinical and experimental settings has shown that doctors treat patients differently in ways that are associated with the patient's gender, race and ethnicity.[44]

As further evidence of racial effects in care and treatment, a number of studies have examined and found racial differences in the treatment of pain, with Whites more likely to be adequately treated for pain than other races and ethnic groups. Some research shows that racial and ethnic minority groups appear to be at a particularly high risk of receiving inadequate treatment for pain in emergency departments. In one study, White patients with pain were more likely to receive an opioid (31 percent) than Black (23 percent), Hispanic (24 percent), or Asian/other patients (28 percent) ($P < .001$ for trend) and differences did not diminish over time.

In my own case, my introduction to this disease state, health crisis and eventual treatment was triggered by pain. I was experiencing persistent, debilitating lower back pain that seemed to outweigh the small fracture in my vertebrae. I consistently presented myself as suffering from pain at the first consultation and throughout my interactions with the chiropractor and the surgeon specializing in pain treatment. I continued to complain of pain during regular and sustained physical therapy with the physical therapist. I am grateful that the blood tests revealed something awry because my reports of pain were not effective at initiating an earnest investigation as to what was wrong.

The healthcare system, like the housing and education infrastructure, represents a well-known social context in which accepted traditions and norms dictate access to resources and rewards. People of color in the United States face barriers to obtaining the quantity and quality of healthcare that White Americans receive. Whether it is in not having sufficient insurance, in navigating the sometimes hostile terrain of the medical system, the biases of healthcare personnel or in experiencing chronic illness that disproportionately impacts poor people, the outcome is the same. Racial minority persons in the United States are less well off, receive less quality care, and are less likely to survive major illnesses than Whites.

44 In one study examining doctors' communication style and interactions with patients, the authors concluded that physicians' encounters with black patients revealed communicative difficulties that may lower quality of care for these patients. See Street Jr., R. L., Gordon, H., & Haidet, P. (2007). Physicians' Communication and Perceptions of Patients: Is it How They Look, How They Talk, or is it Just the Doctor.

A Physician Who Looked Like Me

Ultimately, I decided to consult a MedStar Washington Hospital physician who was a Black woman. I found her only after scrolling through the various websites of multiple hospitals within the area. In doing so, I calculated the likelihood that my interactions with her would not be burdened by the biases and stereotypes that others likely harbored about someone like me. Although I knew nothing else about the doctor but her race and gender, I reasoned that the chances of her seeing me as an individual were greater than they would have been with any one of the other physicians listed, who would inevitably need to spend time getting past any stereotypes and unconscious biases they had about people that looked like me. Not knowing how long this kind of social investigation would go on before they could undertake the task of trying to save my life, I elected to go with the doctor, who, like me, happened to be a Black woman. It is impossible to describe the sense of gratitude I experienced when I contacted her office and was given an appointment within a week's time.

I arrived promptly for my appointment at the MedStar Washington Hospital Center, formerly known as the Washington Hospital Center. It is located in the Northwest section of Washington, D.C., in a neighborhood that has historically been a predominantly Black neighborhood. As such, it has weathered many of the changes that African Americans have collectively endured throughout the last century and now within the first two decades of the twenty-first century. More recently, the neighborhood in which the hospital is located has undergone pockets of gentrification, in which many of the newest homeowners are White professionals working on Capitol Hill and in government and corporate settings. Other long-term residents of the neighborhood, predominantly African Americans, comprise the bulk of the employees who help to run the hospital.

The waiting room at the cancer institute where I came to meet the doctor for the first time, although not packed, had several people waiting there. They were all African Americans who appeared to be in varying stages of sickness and health. Although most of them appeared to be older, they may not have been. There is something about the devastating effects of the disease that finds its way into a person's countenance, making it difficult to accurately detect a person's age.

After waiting for about 30 minutes, I was ushered into an exam room, where the doctor, a tall, brown-skinned woman, entered shortly afterward. She was accompanied by a resident and introduced herself and then the resident, a young woman of color. Originally from the West Indies, "Dr. S" had a melodious accent that reminded me of my own very distant (nearly four generations removed) Caribbean ancestry. I explained my condition to her and what I had learned. The first thing she said to me was that she was so very sorry that I had this disease. It was to be the first (and last) time that any healthcare provider had said this to me. I was grateful for her sympathy.

She told me that there had been remarkable improvement with the drugs that could be used to tackle this disease. Ten years ago, she acknowledged that, this would have been a death sentence with little chance of survival, but with the medicines available today, rates of survival were greatly enhanced. And she had a preliminary plan for me: a rigorous treatment plan involving a drug still considered experimental by some because of its novelty. She promised to follow up with me later that week. I left there feeling encouraged.

Several days later, I heard back from Dr. S. in a phone call that lasted about 30 minutes. She explained to me what the initial treatment would entail and what the likely side effects would be. She answered each of my questions and even volunteered information about things I was uncomfortable asking, like whether I would lose my hair. She told me that, unlike most common cancer treatment drugs, this treatment would not cause me to lose my hair. The treatment plan would be rigorous, initially requiring weekly chemotherapy, with the first infusion beginning later that week. Although she made no promises, she explained that within 6 months, we should expect to achieve remission.

I learned that Dr. S had been engaged in treating patients for this deadly disease for quite some time and was something of an expert in it, as well as another deadly but better-known disease, sickle cell disease. Sickle cell disease, named for the mutated shape of the red blood cell, is caused by the production of abnormal hemoglobin, which binds with other abnormal hemoglobin molecules within the red blood cell to cause rigid deformation of the cell. In the United States it disproportionately affects African Americans and is also observed in people from countries in the Mediterranean, as well as Turkey, the Arabian Peninsula, the Indian subcontinent, and those from the Caribbean, South America, and Central America. Dr. S had acquired experience in treating amyloidosis from working previously at one of the national research and treatment facilities for the disease within the United States, Boston University Medical Center.

Remarkably, although I had yet to begin the arduous plan for treatment and what was to come next, for the first time I felt at ease. The sense of security in knowing that I had identified a doctor who had my best interests at heart and who seemed to be genuinely concerned with my well-being mitigated the stress of my predicament. There were countless other stressors I wrestled with during this time, but being confident about my doctor's intentions for treatment alleviated what had been an overwhelming source of anxiety.

Clearly, there are profound challenges for Black women navigating the healthcare system. In a 2020 blog post for Well+Good, reproductive endocrinologist Nataki Douglas underscores the problem of racism and the lack of providers of color in enumerating the health disparities African American women face in healthcare.[45] In addition to pointing out the necessary changes to the entire medical system, including the problem of implicit bias, she recommends that Black women make changes to the way they engage healthcare providers by documenting everything (their experiences, symptoms, etc.) and putting all of their symptoms in a calendar or diary to show frequency, pain and anything that provided relief.

I believe this to be sound advice. Throughout my consultations, I have tried to personalize my interactions with providers. For example, in asking a doctor for advice or opinion, I try to first ask what they would tell their sister, mother, or friend if they were in a similar position to me. I have found that although this often causes them to pause, they recover pretty quickly and usually provide me with what seems to be a thoughtful response that includes positive and negative aspects of the recommendation. Although I cannot be sure at the time that this is indeed the best advice, I make a note of it and return to it as I consider next steps.

45 See post at https://www.wellandgood.com/black-women-health-care/.

Chapter 3

HEALTH EQUITY AS A PERENNIAL PURSUIT

Despite contemporary vitriol to the contrary, race continues to be a variable that influences interactions among people throughout the United States. Interactions between people of certain races (e.g., Blacks and Whites) are especially likely to be affected. Because of systemic socioeconomic and historical influences, the quality of interracial interactions is often compromised. One can observe some of the most pronounced attenuation in the quality of interactions between African Americans and Whites, and this occurs across all sectors, including healthcare, law enforcement, education and schools, real estate, shops, restaurants, and more.

Ironically, most scientists who study human beings in all of their complexity—from their genomic basis to their cultural traditions—recognize that race as a variable says little about meaningful variations within and across human beings. Indeed, "race" is primarily a visual classifier rather than an indicator of a distinct subspecies of the human population.[1] Instead, its importance lies in its roots as a means for justifying the enslavement and later subjugation of a class of people. Thus, the highly profitable triangular slave trade of Africans and the ensuing system of slavery that enabled the economic growth of the newly established United States required a separation of "races" and inferiorizing of Africans.

Our nation's current reality is tethered to its past, which was built, cultivated, and allowed to flourish on the basis of a racist structure enabled by racist beliefs. For a large part of the time in which the United States has existed, it has either explicitly called for racial separation or implicitly sanctioned racist treatment of its constituents. Of the 245 years of its existence, the United States has only legislated against racist treatment to varying degrees

1 See Montagu, A. (1942). *Man's Most Dangerous Myth: The Fallacy of Race*. New York, NY: Columbia University Press; and Gould, S. J. (1996). *The Mismeasure of Man*. New York, NY: W.W. Norton & Co.

within the last 70 years. Racism is a "multilevel system of oppression based on the social categories of race whereby the superordinate group (traditionally Whites in the United States) subordinates members of other racial groups using overt and covert methods."[2]

> Racism exists at individual, institutional, and cultural levels. Individual racism is interpersonal discrimination; for instance, perpetration of hate crimes against people of color or refusal to rent to an interracial couple.[3] Institutional racism resides in the policies and practices of governments, courts, businesses, schools, etc., to subordinate people of color and benefit white communities. Id. at 141. Although Black people are no longer legally considered three-fifths of a person, the "separate but equal" doctrine is no longer good law, Asians may own land, and Native Americans may now practice their religions, institutional racism continues in disproportionate incarceration rates, discriminatory bank lending practices, racial profiling, environmental racism that allows factories to pollute minority neighborhoods while preserving the purity of wealthier White neighborhoods, de facto housing segregation, and so on. Id. Finally, cultural racism "is the overarching umbrella under which both individual and institutional racism flourish": cultural racism venerates and propagates a worldview in which one group's cultural heritage—White Western Europeans'—is superior to all others.' resulting in the imposition of those "superior" cultural standards upon other groups. Thus, cultural racism is how the legacy of Manifest Destiny became a preference for individualism, capitalism, Christianity, the English language, and Eurocentric beauty standards, all of which persists to this day the legacy of Manifest Destiny became a preference for individualism, capitalism, Christianity, the English language, and Eurocentric beauty standards, all of which persists to this day.[4]

Well-intentioned civil rights policies and legislation that arose in response to collective outcries protesting discrimination prohibited previously acceptable discriminatory behavior. Legislation like *Brown v. Board of Education*, the Civil Rights Act of 1964, and the Voting Rights Act of 1965 struck down what

2 Byrd, W. Carson. (2011). Conflating Apples and Oranges: Understanding Modern Forms of Racism. *Sociology Compass* 5: 1005–1007.

3 Sue, Derald Wing. (2011). Microaggressions in Daily Life, 140–141.

4 Mansoor, H. S. (2019). Modern Racism but Old-Fashioned IIED: How Incongruous Injury Standards Deny "Thick Skin" Plaintiffs Redress for Racism and Ethnoviolence. *Seton Hall Law Review* 50 (3), Article 8. https://scholarship.shu.edu/shlr/vol50/iss3/8.

was previously accepted as racial discrimination in education, employment, and voting. Progress toward reducing racial disparity results from legislation like this.

Ironically, most measures of Americans' internal states and dispositions reveal evidence of lingering motives and feelings that give rise to discrimination and prejudice. Thus, while most Americans openly refute outright prejudice and racial discrimination, implicit measures of their inner states suggest they feel otherwise. It is this psychic conflict resulting from the outward expression of nonracial beliefs coupled with existing racist sentiment that some scholars in this area say gives rise to behavioral instability, which in turn results in racially amplified behaviors.[5]

Today's national conversations are highly politicized, and debates about the role of race in society have catapulted the once little-known framework of critical race theory (CRT) into national discourse, appearing regularly in popular formats like the evening news and talk radio. CRT provides a framework for understanding the insidious and ubiquitous effects of racial discrimination in our society.[6] With CRT, racial discrimination against Black people and other people of color is acknowledged as a cornerstone of American society. Those who protest the veracity of CRT tend to discount the impact of America's racist past, ignore existing systemic racial biases and discrimination, and oppose the teaching of curriculum detailing America's racist past.

Nevertheless, race continues to matter, and, as most scholars who have addressed this contend, until there is sufficient reckoning about the way that it continues to affect people's lives, society will continue to be plagued by racial outrage, discrimination, and unrest. Race differences continue to be responsible for many challenges we currently confront across areas in our multi-racial society. For the different racial groups in America, no interaction seems to matter more than in relationships between Blacks and Whites. The reality of the treacherous historical arrangements that defined relations between Blacks and Whites continues to dictate less than harmonious, sometimes poisonous, relations decades later.

5 Katz, I. (1981). *Stigma: A Social Psychological Analysis.* Hillsdale, NJ: Lawrence Erlbaum; Katz, I., & Hass, R. G. (1988). Racial Ambivalence and American Value Conflict: Correlational and Priming Studies of Dual Cognitive Structures. *Journal of Personality and Social Psychology* 55: 893–905.

6 Delgado, R., Stefancic, J., & Harris, A. (2017). *Critical Race Theory (Third Edition): An Introduction.* New York: New York University; George. (2021). A Lesson in Critical Race Theory.

Healthcare Settings

In healthcare settings, differential race within the doctor-patient interaction can be a barrier. This should not be surprising. Healthcare settings are not immune from the problems arising from racial differences that exist in the criminal justice system, the housing market, the educational system, and beyond. Although the 2003 Institute of Medicine report titled *Unequal Treatment* provided the first comprehensive evidence linking racial health disparities to unequal treatment and care, there is continuing ample evidence of this and its associated effects that appears regularly in publications across a range of areas in the healthcare enterprise.[7] Doctor-patient race correspondence has been examined across many different studies to demonstrate differences for patients who are treated by doctors of the same race compared to those whose doctors were of a different race.

The experience of walking around in my own body for the last 50 years has provided me with enough interactions with physicians to know that some never saw me as anything but a case number who fit the "Black, female" demographic category to which I belong. In healthcare settings, it is not surprising that Black patients would be especially attuned to the nature of their interactions with their doctors. In one study conducted in 2002 that examined the results of the Commonwealth Fund Minority Health Survey, the investigators found that patients who had a choice in the selection of their physician reported greater satisfaction with their physicians than did those who did not have a choice and had physicians who were of different racial status. Race correspondence matters in the doctor-patient relationship, and this is particularly so if you are a patient of color.

Not only do studies relying on patient reports of satisfaction indicate this to be the case, but considerable research exists within the last two decades

---

7 See Simeonova, E. (2013). Doctors, Patients and the Racial Mortality Gap. *Journal of Health Economics* 32 (5): 895–908. https://doi.org/10.1016/j.jhealeco.2013.07.002; Ashton, C. M., Haidet, P., Paterniti, D. A., Collins, T. C., Gordon, H. S., O'Malley, K., Petersen, L. A., Sharf, B. F., Suarez-Almazor, M. E., Wray, N. P., & Street Jr., R. L. (2003, February). Racial and Ethnic Disparities in the Use of Health Services. Bias, Preferences, or Poor Communication? *General Internal Medicine* 18: 146–152; Cooper-Patrick, L., Gallo, J. J., Gonzales, J. J., Vu, H. T., Powe, N. R., Nelson, C., & Ford, D. E. (1999). Race, Gender, and Partnership in the Patient-Physician Relationship. *JAMA* 282 (6): 583–589. https://doi.org/10.1001/jama.282.6.583; Bleich, S. N., Simon, A. E., & Cooper, L. A. (2012). Impact of Patient–Doctor Race Concordance on Rates of Weight-Related Counseling in Visits by Black and White Obese Individuals. *Obesity* 20 (3): 562–570.

that demonstrates the pervasiveness of race differences in health outcomes.[8][9] Across the broad race and ethnic groupings of people within the United States, differences in rates of hypertension and heart disease, cancer, diabetes, and obesity are related to race and ethnic status. Not surprisingly, differences in treatment and survival are also apparent. Consider the well-known difference in breast cancer between Black and White women.[10] While Black women are less likely than White women to have breast cancer, they are more likely than White women to die from it, suggesting an obvious difference in diagnosis and treatment.

Race and ethnic differences in health outcomes are evident in rates of susceptibility to disease that are associated with day-to-day stressors, socioeconomic status, and living conditions. They are also evident in health care access, such that minorities are less likely to have private health insurance than Whites and therefore less likely to seek preventive care. These differences are compounded by the interpersonal dynamics that dictate the way that doctors and patients interact with one another. When the patient and doctor first meet, it is likely that the doctor has some information about the patient. It might simply be their race, gender, and age, along with their condition. In some ways, this normative part of the initial consultation phase, which provides only limited demographic information, ensures that the doctor, no matter how well-intentioned, will rely upon stereotypes in processing information about the patient. For me as a patient, the cognitive default is likely to be whatever stereotype about middle-aged Black women they happen to have. The extent to which their thoughts about the patient they have just met differ from the stereotype will be determined largely by the patient.

My engagement with the healthcare system expanded within a month of my cancer diagnosis. After the initial diagnosis, meeting with Dr. S and commencement of chemotherapy, I learned that the cancer had permanently damaged my kidneys. As evident from the surge in creatinine as well as the rapid drop in hemoglobin, I acquired the additional diagnosis of end-stage renal disease (ESRD). My kidneys had failed, and I would now need to add dialysis to the life-saving medical therapy on which I depended.

8 Thomas A. LaVeist and Amani Nuru-Jeter (2002).
9 See Klonoff, E. (2009).
10 See Smedley et al. (2003).

End-Stage Renal Disease

ESRD represented an entirely different world, a place with a distinctive set of rewards and goals. Being a cancer patient was one thing, but being a dialysis patient was an entirely different one, for which I was even more unprepared. For me, the chronic nature of dialysis treatment seemed to be a separate and worse burden than simply experiencing kidney failure.

With ESRD, the kidneys no longer work as they should in order to meet the body's needs. Like many organs, most people are unaware of their kidneys until they fail to work properly. Kidneys filter waste and excess fluids from the body, which are then excreted in urine. If the kidneys are unable to perform their filtering function, dangerous levels of fluids and toxins are allowed to accumulate in the body. In my case, the amyloid deposits from the amyloidosis had accumulated on my kidneys, causing irreversible damage.

At the suggestion of my father, shortly after the initial diagnosis, I scheduled a full workup and consultation with Boston Medical Center. It, along with the Mayo Clinics, is one of approximately 10 U.S.-based medical facilities that provide advanced treatment and care for amyloidosis. On a weekend in October 2019, I made the journey to the clinic for the two-day consultation. We set out on the day following a chemotherapy appointment, and because my body was still struggling with the cocktail of medicines given to me, I was pretty sick the whole way there.

At the Boston Medical Center, I met with a team of doctors and nurses who were led by Dr. S. A middle-aged Indian woman with a warm bedside manner, Dr. S is a world-renowned researcher and clinician in the treatment of amyloidosis. This was to be a defining experience for me and one that set the bar for my impressions of treatment and subsequent healthcare providers fairly high. The team was engaged, polite, and knowledgeable. They asked me questions and provided me with answers. They also provided me with recommendations for the next steps of treatment.

When I met with one of the team members, the nephrologist, she explained the problems concerning the current state of my kidneys. At that time, it was determined that I had stage 4 kidney disease. She told me that I was at risk of needing to be on dialysis but that there still remained some function. I left there wary but hopeful and returned home to the DC metro area.

Three weeks later, it had come to pass. The level of functioning had deteriorated further, and I was diagnosed with ESRD, stage 5. My estimated glomerular filtration rate (eGFR) was in single digits. GFR (glomerular filtration rate) and it is a key indicator of renal function. eGFR is estimated GFR and is a mathematically derived entity based on a patient's serum creatinine level, age, sex, and race. For most healthy people, an eGFR of 90 mL/min or higher is normal. I was introduced to a nephrologist with whom my oncologist, Dr. S, was acquainted. Because of the increased complexity of my case, it seemed practical to consult a nephrologist who was affiliated with the same facility and who was at least in touch with my cancer doctor. This was my first meeting with Dr. V.

Dr. V, a White woman who was an experienced nephrologist on staff at the hospital, appeared to be in her late 50s, maybe even her early 60s. She was polite in our initial consultation, though not particularly forthcoming. In addition to not providing me with any additional insights, guidance or suggestions, I found her relative lack of affect to be off-putting. Indeed, her attitude toward this life-altering predicament that I was wrestling with was cavalier. On one occasion, I said a lot to her assistant, who relayed some part of my distress to her. Shortly after this, Dr. V followed up with me. That communication lacked any real substance or information, and I can only assume she'd called in response to my message.

I began hemodialysis with one of the two nationally recognized clinics, Fresenius Medical Care (FMC). This entailed showing up at the nearest location, which was about 20 minutes from my home, at scheduled times on three set days each week. I would show up, weigh myself, and then be directed to my assigned dialysis chair, where I was dialyzed for three hours. (This time period would inexplicably change to 3.5–4 hours within two weeks at the clinic.) Once seated, a technician would begin the process of connecting me to a dialysis machine via an access point that had been surgically made below my neck in my chest. The dialyzer was connected to my blood vessel. Because the process entails the movement of blood in and out of the body, it was important to continuously keep track of blood pressure. I would learn that this latter detail would prove to be a challenge. In the first week of doing this, I witnessed a patient whose pressure had dropped so low and so quickly that he had passed out. Paramedics were summoned and responded quickly, successfully reviving the patient.

In my own case, my blood pressure fluctuated considerably, resulting in periodic bouts of unsteadiness, a loss of energy and anxiety every time I sat in the chair. The technicians who assisted me initially at the dialysis clinic differed in terms of their attention to detail. If they were not cognizant of the subtle fluctuations in the readings, I risked a rapid drop in pressure. How much they attended to me determined how I fared on the machine, and I naturally developed a preference for the techs who were particularly alert and engaged. It was a hit-or-miss situation, driven in part by the clinic's staffing roster.

Dialysis in America is a booming business. The population of people receiving dialysis continues to grow, especially in low- and middle-income countries. The global prevalence of kidney failure is uncertain, but it is estimated to be approximately 5.3 million people as recently as 2017.[11] Alternative estimates are as high as 9.7 million.[12] Around the world, millions of people die of kidney failure each year owing to a lack of access to kidney replacement therapy (KRT), often without supportive care.

Throughout my initial engagement with the world of dialysis, I continued to struggle with the reality of my current situation. In addition to the actual act of dialysis, I had to rethink my diet and way of existing. Although I was not a poor eater previously, ESRD meant that I had to be vigilant about specific foods. There were foods I could no longer consume (e.g., sushi, grapefruit), salt was a no-no, and I had to restrict my overall consumption of liquids. This was all very challenging to me, although I knew that I was not alone.

Dialysis has been a growing KRT for the past 50 years, since its emergence in 1972. During the past five decades, how it is delivered and who is able to receive it have changed. Early on, it was limited to well-resourced, Western nations' high-income patients who doctors deemed suitable. Interestingly, it was the process of determining who would receive dialysis that gave rise to the field of bioethics.[13] Issues of fairness instigated valuable discussions and principles about fairness in the receipt of dialysis.

In the early 1970s, dialysis was primarily home hemodialysis. It was a highly specialized therapy limited to approximately 10,000 people in North America and Europe. Following the vivid, live demonstration of a patient being dialyzed in front of the U.S. Congress House Ways and Means Committee in October of 1972, a congressional amendment to the Social Security Act created Medicare entitlement for ESRD. Thus, with the official diagnosis of ESRD, a person is eligible for Medicare at any age.[14]

The provision and availability of dialysis expanded as it moved from highly specialized and limited therapy to a more mainstream healthcare option. Along with the expansion of dialysis came the development of the for-profit outpatient dialysis provider industry. The U.S. kidney dialysis industry

11 Bikbov, B., et al. Global, Regional, and National Burden of Chronic Kidney Disease, 1990–2017: A Systematic Analysis for the Global Burden of Disease Study.

12 Liyanage, T., et al. Worldwide Access to Treatment For End-Stage Kidney Disease: A Systematic Review.

13 Himmelfarb, J., Vanholder, R., Mehrotra, R., et al. The Current and Future Landscape of Dialysis.

14 At 54, I am in the process of applying for Medicare because I have been advised it will be necessary to ensure that all hospital costs for me and a donor will likely exceed what is allowed from my private insurance. I will need Medicare to supplement the payment of these extraordinary costs.

is a huge industry today and is estimated to be worth $24.7 billion in 2018, up 5.5 percent from 2017. The total market is forecasted to grow at a 4 percent average annual pace to $29.7 billion by 2023.[15]

The nearly 7,500 dialysis outpatient centers in the U.S. exist within a very concentrated market. Four industry partners receive 85 percent of the revenue, and two companies control the market: DaVita Partners in the United States and Fresenius Medical Care, which is based in Germany. With similar operating models, the clinics are dominated largely by a small army of technicians who are guided by a registered nurse. A nephrologist shows up periodically to perform a cursory review of patient charts. There is also a nutritionist and a social worker assigned to each shift.

A few months into this new routine that defined my almost surreal existence, I switched dialysis centers. I struggled with the variability in the care I had been receiving from FMC's technicians. In addition, and perhaps more importantly, I did not feel that the nephrologist—Dr. I.—to whom I was now assigned as a patient there had given adequate consideration of my case before assigning me to the 3.5 hours on the machine, which he had seemingly pulled out of the air. Despite my repeated requests for an explanation about why I now needed to stay an additional 30 minutes, Dr. I insisted I maintain the 3.5-hour dialysis session.

While the half-hour difference may not seem like a big deal, it was. My routine was such that I rushed out of work at 5:00 p.m. and arrived at the clinic by 5:30–5:45 p.m. How soon thereafter I got connected depended on the technicians available, and that determined at what time that evening I could be disconnected. I would rush home in time to see my son, who was 11 at the time before he fell asleep for the evening. When Dr. I, who happened to be another Indian man, asked me why the 30 minutes mattered so much, it was clear he thought little of my explanation. Imagine my disappointment when, after switching to another clinic that was part of the DaVita company, I learned that Dr. I also served their patients.

I was stuck, though grateful to have been assigned to the other nephrologist servicing the clinic—Dr. S. Dr. S was also an Indian man and seemed more reasonable than Dr. I. He acknowledged that a three-hour dialysis time would suffice for me.

Three evenings a week, I showed up and underwent dialysis. As I sat in that chair, I took stock of my surroundings. Studying each of the other patients

15 LaRosa, J. (2019). U.S. Kidney Dialysis Clinics Form a Profitable $24 Billion Industry. Downloaded 8/1/202: https://blog.marketresearch.com/u.s.-kidney-dialysis-clinics-form-a-profitable-24-billion-industry.

within sight, I inevitably formed opinions about each of them. A different set of circumstances had propelled each of the approximately 15 other patients who shared my chair shift to need dialysis. For some, it was diabetes or high blood pressure acquired later in life. A considerable number of people were in their middle years, as well as HIV-positive patients across the lifespan. There were any number of pre-existing health factors to which their kidney disease could have been attributed. The patients also differed in terms of their apparent socioeconomic backgrounds. This was evident in that some people necessarily waited patiently for rides to and from the dialysis clinic, compared to others who drove themselves in late-model vehicles.

Yet remarkably, the common thread that united 95 percent of the other patients I observed at the initial FMC clinic and later at the DaVita clinic I moved to was skin color. In both cases, the overwhelming majority of dialysis patients were people of color. They were Black and Brown native-born Americans and immigrants, and although I did not know their individual situations, I knew what foods they should and should not eat, what their relative energy levels were like and where they spent a large part of their time.

Today, one in three Americans is at risk for kidney disease. There are certain risk factors which make ESRD more likely. A constellation of factors makes kidney disease more likely for African Americans, Hispanics, Native Americans, and Asian Americans. More African Americans have kidney disease than any other race/ethnic group.[16] The reason for this has to do with the higher frequency of diabetes and high blood pressure among African Americans, as well as the distinctive way that diabetes affects African Americans.[17]

One indicator of the prevalence of kidney disease among African Americans has to do with the way that eGFR is calculated. As mentioned previously, eGFR, an estimate of how well your kidneys are working, is calculated on the basis of a person's age, sex, and whether or not they are African American, among other things. This highlights the significance of kidney disease among African Americans.

---

16 Eneanya, N. D., Yang, W., & Reese, P. P. (2019). Reconsidering the Consequences of using Race to Estimate Kidney Function. *JAMA* 322: 113–114.

17 Some research describes the way social influences can become embodied, having durable and even transgenerational influences on the most pressing U.S. health disparities. See for example Kuzawa, C. W., & Elizabeth Sweet, E. (2008). Epigenetics and the Embodiment of Race: Developmental Origins of US Racial Disparities in Cardiovascular Health; and Vick, A. D., & Burris, H. H. (2017). Epigenetics and Health Disparities. 7.

The debate in the medical profession continues today about the meaning of racial differences in creatinine levels, which drive apparent differences in GFR. Nevertheless, the "race-corrected" eGFR remains the standard.

In March 2021, the National Kidney Foundation, in partnership with the American Society of Nephrology, issued a joint statement asserting that race modifiers should not be included in equations used to estimate kidney function. Because race is a social construct and not a biological one, it should not be used as an indicator of kidney disease. Instead, current race-based equations should be replaced by an accurate, standardized approach to diagnosing kidney diseases.

This matters because disparities in kidney disease are not limited to differences in prevalence rates. That is, it is not just the case that more African Americans and people of color suffer from kidney disease than do Whites. Unfortunately, health inequities exist in terms of differences in treatment and care, specifically in treatment modality, including access to kidney transplantation. While African Americans represent more than a third (35 percent) of the people receiving dialysis in the United States, they are less likely to be identified as kidney transplant candidates compared to non-Hispanic Whites. I will say more about the transplant process in a later section of this book.

Race as a social variable has shaped the healthcare system and determined access to and availability of treatment and care.[18] In a racially stratified nation in which resources are allocated on the basis of racial status, such as the U.S. healthcare, including medicine, physicians, and other remedies, is delivered in ways reflecting the racial hierarchy. Indeed, because of the disproportionately high representation of African Americans and other people of color with kidney disease requiring dialysis to stay alive, this area of medicine is one that is particularly plagued by the problem of racism. To repeat, racial and ethnic inequities are prolific throughout the healthcare system, and this is especially evident in nephrology.

As an African American woman receiving clinic-based hemodialysis, I was acutely aware of the racial landscape of dialysis—among those requiring it and its healthcare providers. Among the latter, nephrologists, with the exception of Dr. V, most frequently tended to be Indian males. And while they too are part of the larger grouping of people of color, I believe their status as such did little to jeopardize the stability and existence of healthcare inequities.

The context for the delivery of kidney care and treatment of kidney disease is highly racialized, with black and brown patients receiving care from

18 Vyas, D. A., Eisenstein, L. G., & Jones, D. S. (2020). Hidden in Plain Sight — Reconsidering the Use of Race Correction in Clinical Algorithms.

Indian and White doctors. The delivery of care for hemodialysis patients takes place in the structured, closed space of the dialysis clinic. Patients are treated politely but with little regard for the distinctive attributes that define them. Perhaps that is appropriate and contributes to efforts to balance the quality of care.

Nevertheless, in my case, I found myself frequently needing to remind the technicians and the nurse on duty that I was employed (accounting for why I arrived at a time that coincided with my departure from a senior position in a 9–5 job) and that I had specific reasons for wanting to come off of the machine that were associated with my status as a mom of a school-aged child. For these reasons alone, I was unlike everyone else.

Most patients on kidney dialysis are unemployed. This is a vexing issue that appears worldwide. Employment rates in the United States for patients on dialysis are disapprovingly low.[19] Patients with ESRD face many barriers to remaining in or joining the workforce after starting dialysis. These include poor employment opportunities because of lower socioeconomic status, fatigue, and other symptoms of renal failure, depression and feelings of social isolation, comorbid diseases, transportation issues, potential loss of disability and/or medical assistance benefits with employment, scheduling conflicts with dialysis, and the assumption by some employers that patients on dialysis are too sick or undependable to work. Rounding out all of these factors is the societal perception that people with ESRD are unable to work. Thus, it is not at all surprising that a majority of ESRD patients are unemployed.[20]

There are various wrap-around services that kidney patients can pursue to help with any one of the barriers identified earlier, but they exist piecemeal, and it is primarily up to the patient to pursue them. Services like nutritional and psychological counseling, metro access and financial assistance exist for dialysis patients, but for many patients, the effort to engage them is akin to the effort in working in actual paid employment.

Early on, during the initial stages of kidney disease, my father accompanied me to an appointment with Dr. V to discuss the need for dialysis and to consider the options for doing this. I had heard about the home dialysis process, which a minority of patients managed at home, and I was interested in the possibility of doing this. I was starting from ground zero in that I knew nothing about what these forms of home dialysis involved, but I was anxious for an option other than the kidney center one.

---

19 Hallab, A., & Wish, J. B. (2018). Employment among Patients on Dialysis. An Unfulfilled Promise. *Clinical Journal of the American Society for Nephrology*.

20 Kutner, N., Bowles, T., Zhang, R., Huang, Y., & Pastan, S. (2008). Dialysis Facility Characteristics and Variation in Employment Rates: A National Study.

This would be my second time meeting face-to-face with Dr. V, who was affiliated with the MedStar Washington hospital system. Extremely busy, she made it clear that she had limited time to spend with us, and my father and I were necessarily pressured to be concise and succinct. She was polite and did her best, it seemed to answer my questions. However, it became clear midway through this conversation that Dr. V would be challenged to envision an individualized course of therapy for me. Instead, she lumped me into the category in which she held all (or most) of her dialysis patients. This became evident as I expressed problems with the shift schedule at the clinic and my ability to get there following work.

I told her that I wanted to know more about possible home dialysis options, which could alleviate the stress of having to rush to the clinic at the end of the workday. In responding to me, she first began with a lecture about the federal government's decision to make dialysis eligible for Medicare. She explained that because I had kidney disease, I could now go on disability. Her eyes lit up as she described this option to me. "You'll just have to stop working," she matter-of-factly concluded.

My father and I both responded audibly, saying, "No, this wasn't my preferred course. It was not an option I was interested in pursuing." It was difficult for me not to become emotional as I impressed upon her my desire to keep working. More than the income it generated, my work and its accompanying accomplishments defined a large part of my identity. That identity was currently under assault. I was no longer the person I understood myself to be some months earlier. This health crisis had permanently altered my vision of myself. In addition to its impacts on my physical appearance, which included significant weight loss and a darkening of my complexion and skin tone, it had also impacted my self-perception of my appearance along with my self-esteem. The prospect of further altering my identity by no longer working at this stage of my life was far more than I could imagine handling. I made it clear that I was determined to keep working.

Ultimately, I decided upon the home dialysis method called peritoneal dialysis for kidney failure. With peritoneal dialysis (PD) as it is commonly referred to, the patient's peritoneum (in the abdomen) is used as a filter to remove toxins, correct electrolyte balance, and remove excess fluids. In peritoneal dialysis, the inside lining of your own belly acts as a natural filter. Wastes are taken out by means of a cleansing fluid called dialysate, which is washed in and out of your belly in cycles.[21] A small plastic catheter is inserted into the abdomen, and sterile cleansing fluid is inserted and then removed.

21 National Kidney Foundation. Downloaded https://www.kidney.org/atoz/content/peritoneal, August 11, 2021.

Dr. V referred me to a surgeon within the hospital who was highly regarded and performed the catheter insertion for PD.

My first step toward PD involved a consultation with the surgeon, Dr. H. I showed up for the appointment a few minutes early, accompanied by my father. The tiny waiting room was packed. Indeed, because there were not enough seats, we eyed enviously the other patients who had arrived before us and were seated. Eventually, as patients were called and went behind closed doors, the waiting area began to empty out and we were able to sit while waiting. Eventually, after nearly 50 minutes of waiting, my name was called and we went in.

Dr. H greeted us warmly, shaking hands and smiling before indicating where we should sit. Of Middle Eastern descent, he appeared to be in his late 50s or early 60s. A slim build, his hair was long and secured in a ponytail.

He spoke softly and directly, making eye contact. For PD, part of the consultation involves the surgeon's informal assessment of the patient's physical and psychological ability to successfully manage the dialysis procedure. I was aware that he was not only listening to my answers to his questions but also implicitly evaluating my suitability for PD. Not everyone can manage the requirements of PD, and all PD patients run the risk of peritonitis. Peritonitis is a serious infection of the abdomen that is an occasional complication and can eliminate the use of the peritoneum for future dialysis.

After about 25 minutes, we concluded our conversation, agreeing to proceed with the next steps. He informed me that a member of his staff would be following up with a date for surgery. He had agreed to perform the surgery to insert the catheter into my abdomen. Three weeks later, the surgery, performed on an outpatient basis, was successfully completed. I came home with a 6-inch small plastic tube protruding from a small hole and securely taped to my abdomen, with strict instructions to avoid getting wet.

Two weeks later, I met with the PD nurse at another DaVita clinic. The clinic where I had gone for hemodialysis did not have PD available, and I had scheduled this appointment several weeks earlier. My husband accompanied me to the initial appointment with Nurse J. Nurse J was a petite, mature woman from the Philippines whom I would come to know quite well. However, on day one, I was unprepared for the weight of what the daily burden of PD entails, and as she introduced us to the process, I once again found myself struggling to cope with this new reality. The nurse sympathized with me, pausing to think of kind things to say. I was required to have two-weeks of PD training before I could manage the process on my own. That meant I would need to continue visiting the other clinic for the three-times-a-week hemodialysis sessions in addition to my near-daily visits to the PD clinic. It seemed overwhelming.

At the end of the training, nurse J, accompanied by another nurse I had never met before, came to my home. She had a checklist of items to go over with me as the equipment required for PD was delivered and installed. After about an hour of walking me through the process once again and reminding me of the necessary details, they left. I began PD on the automatic cycler that evening, and now, more than a year later, I have been conducting it every evening since that time.

There are two types of PD: continuous ambulatory PD (CAPD) and automated PD (APD). The latter uses a machine, called the cycler, that delivers and then drains the cleansing fluid for the patient. Most people perform this treatment at night while sleeping. The other kind of P.D. is done while the patient engages in their other normal activities—while working, eating, watching television, etc. With CAPD, the treatment is performed by placing about two quarts of cleansing fluid into the abdomen and later draining it. After an exchange (putting in and taking out the fluid) is completed, the discarded fluid (which now has waste removed from your blood) is drained from the patient and thrown away. This 30–40 minute process is usually done three, four or five times in a 24-hour period during normal activities.

I am well aware of the burden of PD. I am also very much aware of its life-sustaining value. Because of the impact of amyloidosis on my kidneys, I could not survive without dialysis. I have elected to use PD because it allows me to continue living relatively normally. I continue to serve as a chauffeur for many of my son's activities, I work in a fairly demanding job as a senior executive, and remain actively engaged in all manner of activities associated with being a wife and mother.

My health crisis began before the COVID-19 pandemic swept across the United States. At the time, I was just becoming familiar with the process of hemodialysis and incorporating the multiple weekly visits into my routine. The virus' impact was just beginning to take shape. One evening at the clinic during this time, the social worker made a point of providing each of the patients with a note on the clinic's letterhead indicating ESRD status and the need for dialysis. It represented a "pass" in the event that any one of us were stopped by the police because a curfew had recently been implemented. By the time our dialysis session ended and we were disconnected, a small number of us left the clinic to travel home during the time period of the official curfew. The note was meant to explain our reasons for being out at that time. During that time, the streets were dark and empty, and I was fortunate not to be accosted by the police.

The intensity and alarm surrounding the virus impacted many of the policies of dialysis clinics nationwide. They were constantly adapting their own protocols to align with the perceived risk of the coronavirus at any one time. The staff had always masked and wore gloves while connecting and disconnecting patients from the blood-purifying dialysis equipment, but the virus extended the masking requirement to everyone, including patients, all of the time, and it now led clinics to prohibit all visitors. Before the virus took hold, during my very first visits to the clinic, my father often accompanied me as much for support as to communicate with the technicians to ensure my well-being. This was no longer permissible.

The dialysis clinic is a high-risk environment for COVID-19 because patients must receive dialysis regardless of their status and because of the greater vulnerability of people with kidney disease to the virus. According to the Centers of Disease Control and Prevention, dialysis patients are at high risk for serious illness and death from COVID-19, and people on dialysis who get COVID-19 have a 50 percent hospitalization rate and a 20–30 percent mortality rate.[22] Patients must receive dialysis whether or not they have been vaccinated, or, as was the case in the early days of the pandemic, whether or not they test positive for the virus.

At that time, I was anxious about completing the training to begin peritoneal dialysis. Although the prospect of carrying out this important life-saving function on my own was daunting, I welcomed the opportunity to remain home and reduce my risk of contracting the virus. My decision and ultimate shift to PD were extraordinarily timely.

At the time of this writing, I am looking forward to being a candidate for kidney transplantation. For many cancer patients, such as myself, there is a window of time for remission required before eligibility. I am waiting and praying to get past that period.

In the meantime, I take stock of the costs of dialysis, shaking my head each month. Of course, it doesn't matter what kind of dialysis we're talking about, they are all expensive. For most patients, the federal government pays 80 percent of all dialysis charges, while private insurance or state medical assistance pays the rest. That said, it is difficult to reconcile the costs included on the statements I periodically receive for dialysis.

Each month I receive an itemized accounting of the charges DaVita requests payment for along with the allowed reimbursement. Each day within a month, DaVita charges an estimated $10,000, so that the end of the month results in a grand total of about $300,000. I continue to see Nurse J every other week and the nephrologist of the clinic to whom I assigned about once a month. I perform PD on my own each evening and reorder and receive supplies once a month. I am using a refurbished machine that DaVita provided me. And still, it is $10,000 each day.

---

22 Centers for Disease Control and Prevention, https://www.cdc.gov/vaccines/covid-19/planning/dialysis-partners-jurisdictions.html, Downloaded August 12, 2021.

Chapter 4

THE SUBTLETY OF SKIN TONE BIAS AND RACISM IN ACCESS TO QUALITY CARE

As a result of the cumulative effects of the illness and noticeable weight loss, my appearance changed in yet another way. Whereas my complexion had previously been "light," it was now somewhere closer to a medium, darker brown color. I was frustrated when I first noticed this because no one, not even Dr. S., the African American physician who currently treats me, could tell me that this was a direct result of amyloidosis or multiple myeloma, or that it was a direct result of kidney failure, or that it was some kind of outcome resulting from the cumulative effects of these maladies. Even now, some 20 months into the diagnosis, I continue to struggle with a true understanding of the effects on my complexion. I regularly grapple with any number of unanswerable questions. For example, will my skin tone continue to get darker with additional treatment? Alternatively, will sufficient treatment reverse these effects? Will my skin tone return to the shade it once was?

For me, as an African American woman in a racialized society like the United States, the matter of skin color (i.e., complexion) is very real. While I was aware of my shifting skin tone and noticed it most times when I looked in the mirror, I did not become sensitive to the change until greeting my mother at the airport after not having seen her for close to a year. She actually gasped and stopped in her tracks as she approached me, immediately questioning whether something was wrong. My mother, who has always had a medium brown skin tone, immediately sensed something was off given the change in my skin tone.

This was nearly a year before I would be diagnosed with amyloidosis/multiple myeloma. Unbeknownst to me, the disease was progressing largely undetectably. Whereas others who saw me daily did not notice the change in my skin tone, my mother, who lives outside of the United States and who had not seen me in months, noticed the change right away. I was not terribly alarmed, but I did become concerned.

It would be several months before I saw a doctor, a general practitioner. The doctor happened to be an Indian American man. At our first consultation, I mentioned the change in my skin tone to him when he asked whether I had noticed any physical differences or changes. It is hard to say what he thought about this because he did not respond to this detail. He looked at me perhaps a few seconds longer than he would have otherwise done and resumed his completion of the intake forms. I asked whether the change in skin tone indicated that something was awry, but he provided me with no answer.

You may be wondering how I let that go without pressing for an answer. Looking back, I think that more than anything, my failure to insist on an answer from the doctor at that point stemmed from my underlying belief that the doctor simply did not know, as well as my implicit desire to avoid making him feel uncomfortable about his inadequacy. That is, I was pretty darn sure he had no real clue about what was going on with me, and I did not wish to embarrass him by pointing that out. So, I let it slide.

It is a curious matter, this skin tone thing.

Today,[1] society's preference for light skin complexions over darker ones remains a persistent and repugnant reminder of the roots of the Black experience in America.[2] Africans brought to the "new world" beginning in the 1600s were enslaved and brutalized by their European captors. The success of the slave system necessitated the development of the belief in racial differences, which over time came to associate race with skin color. Black people and people with darker skin tones occupied the lowest rungs on the social and economic ladder. White people and those with light skin tones were positioned on the higher rungs of the ladder. They possessed greater status overall and controlled all of the resources (e.g., means of production).

White slave owners used skin tone as a dimension of status on their plantations so that slaves with darker skin tones had more onerous jobs and were subjected to more deplorable conditions than were slaves with lighter skin tones. A number of historians have written about slave owners' role in creating another caste of workers.[3] Primarily through brutal force, slave owners often impregnated female slaves who gave birth to children who were enslaved but who appeared lighter in skin tone than most Africans. The offspring of slave

1 Wilson, Russell & Hall. (2013). The Color Complex: The Politics of Skin Color in a New Millennium.

2 Hunter, M. (2007). The Persistent Problem of Colorism: Skin Tone, Status, and Inequality.

3 See Hodes, Martha. (1997). *White Women, Black Men: Illicit Sex in the Nineteenth-Century South*. New Haven: Yale University Press.

owners and their female slaves were called mulattoes, and their growing presence expanded the bounds of racial hierarchy.

By the time slavery ended in the middle of the nineteenth century, the racial hierarchy privileging White landowners had been firmly developed. Those who were White but poor or foreign-born came next in the social hierarchy, followed by people of color in descending order of blackness. That is, people with the darkest skin tones occupied the lowest rung on the social hierarchy.

By the turn of the nineteenth century, it was well established in Black America that people with lighter skin tones had greater resources and life potential, as demonstrated in their educational attainment, where they worked, and how much money they made. Patterns of interaction among African Americans also reflected their skin tones.[4] Those with lighter complexions generally affiliated with one another and with those who had more education, better jobs, and lived in better homes and neighborhoods.[5] Those who descended from mulattoes came from enslaved African women and their White captors, whereas those with darker complexions descended from African women and men without the influence of their captors' ancestry. Their skin tones did not reflect the miscegenation that the skin tones of mulattoes and lighter complexioned Blacks did.

As the United States developed its racialized narrative to support White domination and privilege, the preference for lighter skin tones continued to grow, and today there remains a continued preference for light skin tones.[6,7] This preference has been exported around the world, and it appears to be correlated with European colonization, such that along with the history of colonization throughout the world, there is a global tendency to prefer lighter skin tones.[8] In Asia, Africa, and South America people value lighter skin tones over darker ones.[9] True, there are many "break though" examples of darker skinned Blacks who are highly revered with numerous resources, but the preference and privilege associated with light skin tones remain in the Black community and sadly throughout the diaspora.

---

4 See the book *Skin Deep: Race and Complexion in the Color-Blind Era.*

5 Wirth, L., & Goldhamer, H. (1944). Characteristics of the American Negro; and see Frazier, E. F. (1957). Black Bourgeoisie.

6 Wilson, Russell & Hall (2013).

7 Monk, E. P. (2021). The Unceasing Significance of Colorism: Skin Tone Stratification in the United States; and Jordan, W. (1968). White Over Black.

8 Rondilla, J., & Spickard, P. (2007). Is Lighter Better?

9 Jones, V. (2004). Pride or Prejudice? A Formally Taboo Topic Among Asian-Americans and Latinos Comes Out Into the Open as Skin Tone Consciousness Sparks a Backlash.

Most Black people are loath to acknowledge this.[10] Indeed, during my career as an academic, I spent several rewarding years on the faculty at one of America's largest historically Black universities. It is a place that has educated many of our nation's "first Black" contributors to the arts, science, medicine, and politics. There is an almost palpable sense of Black pride one senses on the campus of that renowned university. Yet, at the very same time, in the very same spaces, one can easily come upon evidence of the continued preference for lighter skin. The bias for light skin tones is nestled alongside the more vocal echoes of Black pride.

Skin tone differences are not simply a matter of conversation or commentary. Unfortunately, society's reactions to skin tone differences among African Americans have resulted in continued differences in wages between light- and dark-skinned African Americans. Research shows that as darkness increases and Afrocentric appearance increases, so does the probability of being perceived as dangerous, incompetent, ugly, and much more.[11] In an example of this, one study found that workers with darker skin tones had lower wages,[12] confirming the hypothesis of a preference for whiteness. That study is not alone, and others reflect similar trends showing that skin color stratifies occupational status.[13] Although there exists an interesting mix of sentiments about skin color in the wider population today, there is continuing evidence of Whites' preference for light-skinned Blacks

Interestingly, skin tone for African Americans often gets wrapped up in perceptions about their affiliation with other Black people. In her edited text Color Matters,[14] law professor Kimberly Jade Norwood describes the practice of "Black think" to describe another way that Blacks are victimized. With Black think, African Americans who do not behave as others (usually other Black people) expect them to are vilified. They are perceived to be disloyal and not authentically Black enough because they make choices, express certain viewpoints and reside in certain neighborhoods that do not align with a majority of Black people. Consider the outpouring of commentary surrounding President Barack Obama and the members of his administration who were appointed. Some people even debated whether Obama, who has a light skin tone, was black enough to fully represent African Americans.

---

10 Hunter, M. (2007). The Persistent Problem of Colorism: Skin Tone, Status, and Inequality.

11 Maddox, K. B. (2004). Perspectives on Racial Phenotypicality Bias.

12 Goldsmith, A. H., Hamilton, D., & Darity, W. Jr. (2007). From Dark to Light: Skin Color and Wages among African-Americans.

13 Monk, E. P. (2014). Skin Tone Stratification among Black Americans, 2001–2003.

14 Norwood, K. J. (2014). Color Matters.

Many people endorse the erroneous belief that African Americans with darker skin tones are more authentically Black.[15] Of course, what that means depends on the content of their beliefs about Black people.[16,17] Across a number of earlier studies, research in social psychology has shown that African Americans with darker skin tones are penalized relative to those with lighter skin tones in a variety of social situations, including the family, educational settings, and prospective marriage partners.[18] Furthermore, research has also shown that darker skin tones are associated with less favorable voter evaluations,[19] less leniency in the criminal justice system[20] including prison time for female offenders,[21] teacher's judgments of students,[22] and more.

---

15 Maddox, K., & Gray, S. A. (2002). Cognitive Representations of Black Americans: Reexploring the Role of Skin Tone. *Personality and Social Psychology Bulletin* 28 (2): 250–259. https://doi.org/10.1177/0146167202282010. And see Hagiwara, N., Kash, D. A., & Cesario, J. (2012). The Independent Effects of Skin Tone and Facial Features on Whites' Affective Reactions to Blacks. *Journal of Experimental Social Psychology* 48 (4): 892–898.

16 Donovan, R. A. (2011). Tough or Tender: (Dis)similarities in White College Students" Perceptions of Black and White Women. *Psychology of Women Quarterly* 35: 458–468. https://doi.org/10.1177/0361684311406874.

17 Lemons, J. S. (1977). Black Stereotypes as Reflected in Popular Culture, 1880–1920. *American Quarterly* 29 (1): 102–116.

18 Drake, St. Clair, & Cayton, Horace R. (1962). *Black Metropolis*. New York: Harper and Row; Freeman, Howard E., Armor, David, Ross, J. Michael, & Pettigrew, Thomas F. (1966). Color Gradation and Attitudes among Middle-Income Negroes. *American Sociological Review* 31: 365–375; Powell-Hopson, Darlene, and Hopson, Derek S. (1988). Implications of Doll Color Preferences among Black Preschool Children and White Preschool Children. *The Journal of Black Psychology* 14: 57–63; Ransford, H. Edward. (1970). Skin Color, Life Chances, and Anti-White Attitudes. *Social Problems* 18: 164–179.

19 Terkildsen, N. (1993). *American Journal of Political Science* 37 (4): 1032–1053; Caliendo, S. M., & Mcilwain, C. D. (2006). Minority Candidates, Media Framing, and Racial Cues in the 2004 Election. *The Harvard International Journal of Press/Politics* 11: 45–69.

20 Blair, I. V., Judd, C. M., & Chapleau, K. M. (2004). The Influence of Afrocentric Facial Features in Criminal Sentencing. *Psychological Science*; Eberhardt, J. L., Goff, P. A., Purdie, V. J., & Davies, P. G. (2004). Seeing Black: Race, Crime, and Visual Processing. *Journal of Personality and Social Psychology* 87 (6): 876–893. https://doi.org/10.1037/0022-3514.87.6.876.

21 Viglione, J., Hannon, L., & DeFina, R. (2011). The Impact of Light Skin on Prison Time for Black Female Offenders.

22 Hughes, B., & Hertel, M. (1990). The Significance of Color Remains: A Study of Life Chances, Mate Selection, and Ethnic Consciousness among Black Americans. *Social Forces* 68: 1105–1120.

As for myself, although I recognized that skin tone bias, or "colorism," can be complex[23]—simultaneously providing advantages or disadvantages depending on the social context, as my illness progressed, I became increasingly sensitive to others' perceptions of me and treatment of me associated with my now increasingly darker skin tone. Whereas many people remain unaware of their own preferences for lighter skin tones, I was very much aware of the privileged position my pre-disease lighter skin tone afforded me. After my illness, I experienced the world as someone with a darker skin tone. As much as it was possible, I realized my own complicity in the perpetuation of light skin privilege at the very same time that I forfeited that privilege.

According to sociologist Hunter, who has studied and written extensively about colorism,[24] most of the social science research on skin-tone discrimination focuses on the employment experiences of African Americans and Hispanics.[25] For example, in one study that focused on Hispanics, researchers found a clear hierarchy with white Hispanics at the top, "others" in the middle, and black Hispanics at the bottom. White Hispanics also had lower unemployment rates and lower poverty rates than black Hispanics.[26] In another study that compared the employment experiences of Mexicans, Puerto Ricans, and Cubans in the United States, the researchers found that Mexicans and Cubans with darker skin tones had significantly lower occupational prestige scores than their lighter-skinned counterparts even when controlling for factors that influenced performance in the labor market.[27]

When I considered the volume of research, anecdotal reports and biographies attesting to the way that colorism operates on a day-to-day basis, I was overwhelmed. Each time I looked into the mirror and saw the brown-faced woman staring back at me, I was terrified for her. Although the transformation in skin tone which I experienced was not nearly as noticeable as John Griffin's 1959 intentional transformation into a Black man, it struck me nonetheless. In his classic text Black Like Me, author John Griffin, a White man,

---

23 Russell, K., Wilson, M., & Hall, R. (1992). *The Color Complex*. New York: Doubleday.

24 Hunter, Margaret. (2005). *Race, Gender, and the Politics of Skin Tone*. New York: Routledge.

25 As examples, see: Gomez, Christina. (2000). The Continual Significance of Skin Color: An Exploratory Study of Latinos in the Northeast. *Hispanic Journal of Behavioral Sciences* 22: 94–103. Hughes & Hertel 1990; Hunter, Margaret. (2002). If You're Light, You're Alright: Light Skin Color as Social Capital for Women of Color. *Gender & Society* 16: 175–193.

26 Fears, Darryl. (2003). Race Divides Hispanics, Report Says; Integration and Income Vary With Skin Color. *Washington Post*, July 14, 2003.

27 Espino, Rodolfo, & Franz, Michael. (2002). Latino Phenotypic Discrimination Revisited: The Impact of Skin Color on Occupational Status. *Social Science Quarterly* 83: 612–623.

describes his intentional transformation from that of a White man to a Black man. His transformation was total and shocking, and in his case, the man who looked back at him from the mirror was wholly unrecognizable.

As an African American woman with a newly acquired brown skin tone, my experience was far less dramatic than that of Griffin. That said, I knew that because of my skin tone, I would need to be prepared for an entirely new range of reactions and treatments by others. I anticipated both subtle and direct expressions of discrimination. My greatest concerns were with how I would be regarded and treated by members of the healthcare system. I felt the weight of this additional angst, which only served to exacerbate the distress resulting from my experience with a rare, acute disease that had compromised my kidneys.

Ironically, I realized that now, more than ever before, others would perceive me to be more authentically Black than they had ever done before. Research and anecdotal reports reveal that Black and Whites draw inferences about African Americans' allegiance and identity with "Blackness" based on their skin tone. Many view darker skin tones as more authentically ethnic.[28] Black people with darker skin tones are perceived to be more authentically Black.[29]

This matters in the context of seeking critical health care because of the persistence of negative stereotypes about African Americans and other people of color. From the outset, I felt the burden of being a woman of color as I navigated the various healthcare settings. Dealing with physicians and other healthcare personnel who saw me as an outsider and associated me with any number of stereotypes they had about Black women was frustrating and tiring. But now, as a Black woman with a dark skin tone, I felt the weight and sting of those primarily negative beliefs about me more acutely.

My feelings were not unique or unfounded. As one author notes, "studies also reveal skin tone stratification in health among African Americans. On one hand, skin tone is significantly associated with perceived discrimination among African Americans and given that perceived discrimination is a well-known risk factor for poorer mental and physical health, skin tone plays at least an indirect role in shaping health inequalities among African Americans."[30]

---

28 Hunter, Margaret. (2005). *Race, Gender, and the Politics of Skin Tone.* New York: Routledge.

29 It should be noted that this was not something I had considered previously. Nor had I ever sensed that my light skin tone had compromised my "blackness."

30 See Monk, Ellis P. (2021). The Unceasing Significance of Colorism: Skin Tone Stratification in the United States. *Daedalus* 150 (2): 76–90.

I would go a step further and argue that there are direct effects of skin tone on health too. Consider one study that found evidence that skin tone bias differentiates health among siblings in families.[31] That study used the National Longitudinal Study of Adolescent to Adult Health (Add Health), a nationally representative, longitudinal study of adolescents in grades 7–12 in the fall of 1994 to the spring of 1995 academic year. The researchers used measures of interviewer-reported skin tone to predict ever having been diagnosed with hypertension in Wave IV (self-reported in 2008) when respondents were about 24–32 years old. Findings supported the hypothesis that darker skin tones were more often associated with hypertension, that is, skin tone significantly predicted hypertension outcomes among African Americans and Hispanics. More specifically, they found that each unit's darker complexion—for example, going from medium brown to dark brown—was associated with an increase in the probability of ever having been diagnosed with hypertension.

In my case, understanding better just how the disease's progression was affecting my skin tone would have been better. Having some input from any one of the physicians and specialists I consulted with would have gone a long way in helping me throughout this experience. Unfortunately, this was not the case.[32]

As luck would have it, my father, having worked for decades with dialysis patients, was most capable of explaining what had occurred with my skin tone. First off, he attributed my change in skin tone to kidney failure, rather than amyloidosis or multiple myeloma. Of course, these disease states were in turn responsible for the kidney failure. But in terms of a direct cause for the wholesale darkening of my skin, he was pretty confident it was the kidney failure. As he explained it, the darkening in the skin tone of a patient with end-stage renal disease (ESRD), is believed to occur as a result of several possible metabolic factors. Most likely, the body's balance (or imbalance) of fluids is key. One of those fluids that is out of balance is called bile. The body's automatic response to sensing overload or too much of anything is to get rid of it in any way it can. This can mean pushing it out of the skin. When bile comes to the surface of the skin or just below it, light from the sun, air, pollution, or anything else causes it to darken.

31 Laidley, Thomas, Domingue, Benjamin, Sinsub, Piyapat, et al. (2019). New Evidence of Skin Color Bias and Health Outcomes Using Sibling Difference Models: A Research Note. *Demography* 56 (2): 753–762.

32 Laidley, T., Domingue, B., Sinsub, P., Mullan Harris, K., & Conley, D. (2019). New Evidence of Skin Color Bias and Health Outcomes Using Sibling Difference Models: A Research Note. *Demography* 56: 753–762. DOI: https://doi.org/10.1007/s13524-018-0756-6.

None of the nephrologists with whom I spoke to or consulted with had much to say about this, and my impression is that the change in skin tone I acknowledged experiencing was regarded as little more than a matter of cosmetics. Perhaps if I had been a White woman who suddenly plummeted into the ranks of colored people, my questions would have merited a more spirited response. It is hard to say.

My point in writing about this aspect of my health crisis is to underscore the way that the color of my skin tone, though immeasurably important in contemporary arrangements and interactions, was ignored by virtually all of the medical personnel I consulted with. For some, it may have been that they just didn't see what difference it made—I appeared to be a Black woman before, so what if I was a somewhat darker Black woman? For others, they simply may not have wished to deal with the matter of skin tone and the sensitivities surrounding it.

Perhaps more than any other issue, that of skin tone highlights the value of employing an intersectional approach to better understand the problem of health disparities. Intersectionality is an increasingly popular way of understanding the overall impact of the multiple marginalized statuses that a person holds. It affords an understanding of the interactive effects of a person's gender, race, ethnicity, age, socioeconomic status and more. In the context of health care, an intersectional approach is particularly illuminating. Consider the work by Bowleg (2012),[33] who argues for an intersectional perspective in public health. She describes the way that individual identities and the social inequalities associated with them can lead to health disparities at the institutional level. To fully understand the interactive effects of these dynamics requires researchers and health practitioners to reconceptualize health disparities in ways that reflect the complexity of the population.

It is in this vein that Workman calls for an intersectionality approach, taking account of compounded oppressions, in examining the barriers to kidney transplantation.[34] In the beginning of my illness, I never imagined that I would be in need of transplantation in the future, but I understand now that my future (if I am lucky) will involve transplantation. Unfortunately, this

---

33 Bowleg, Lisa. (2012). The Problem With the Phrase Women and Minorities: Intersectionality—an Important Theoretical Framework for Public Health. Accepted: February 20, 2012. Published Online: June 07, 2012. https://ajph.aphapublications.org/doi/10.2105/AJPH.2012.300750.

34 Workman, K. (2021). Using an Intersectionality Framework to Examine Disparities in the Steps to Kidney Transplantation in Patients with End Stage Renal Disease. University of Richmond: Honors Thesis. https://scholarship.richmond.edu/cgi/viewcontent.cgi?article=2574&context=honors-theses.

process and the decision-making that determines whether a patient is eligible for transplant are anything but transparent.

The paper by Workman presents some sobering insights into this process. The United States continues to allocate resources and provide opportunities on the basis of race, ethnicity, gender, and socioeconomic status. It is not surprising that decisions about transplantation, who receives them and when, are also driven by the value associated with these factors. An intersectionality framework starts from the perspective of acknowledging this reality. Following that, decisions about healthcare and its delivery are informed by specific considerations associated with the individual patient. Thus, if the patient is a single mother, organizing appointments around her childcare availability can be critical. Similarly, patients who perceive racial discrimination are going to be less likely to engage regularly with providers, and that needs to be accounted for in tailoring a treatment schedule for them.

In our increasingly multi-racial society, the relative importance of skin tone increases. It matters more than it once did, and more than race now does. In this context, skin tone is more than a physical trait reflective of value-neutral bodily differences. It is a social construct that is hierarchical in nature and laden with racial bias, stereotypes, and social standing.[35] In one analysis of data from the Life-Course Influences on Fetal Environments (LIFE) study, a retrospective cohort study administered between June 2009 and December 2011, the researchers found differences in the timing of prenatal care associated with reports of racial microaggressions. More microaggressions were associated with delayed prenatal care among African American women at either end of the color continuum, including those who indicated a dark brown as well as a light brown skin tone. The researchers concluded that skin tone-based mistreatment, in tandem with racial discrimination in the form of racial microaggressions, may influence African American women's use of prenatal care.

So far in this chapter, I have discussed the way that skin tone bias disadvantages people of color, and in particular African Americans, across multiple sectors. I have provided evidence of the effects of skin tone bias in healthcare settings and suggested its continuing impact. Using my own experiences as a Black woman with a light skin tone and now a darker brown skin tone, I have tried to describe the way that skin tone operates as another potential barrier to quality care for people of color. I have also suggested the likelihood of its

---

35 Slaughter-Acey, J. C., Sneed, D., Parker, L., & Keith, V. M. (2019). Skin Tone Matters: Racial Microaggressions and Delayed Prenatal Care. *American Journal of Preventive Medicine* 57 (3): 321–329.

increasing importance in our society as the United States becomes increasingly multi-racial.[36]

I think it is important to make a distinction between discrimination stemming from racial prejudice and discrimination stemming from the application of the rule of conditional probability. It is the latter about which I am most concerned and which I believe causes as much harm as the beliefs and actions of devout racists. In this case, the physician may correctly recognize the prevalence of a disease that disproportionately occurs in minority populations, but their knowledge about prevalence crowds out more accurate information about the individual minority person who is their patient. This distinction allows for the recognition that most physicians do not wish to harm their patients.

Initial Treatment for Kidney Disease

After determining that my kidneys were no longer functioning, I underwent a short surgery to insert a subclavian catheter to enable immediate hemodialysis (HD). The subclavian artery supplies oxygen-rich blood to the two sides of the body. This treatment for kidney failure is a process in which the blood is filtered outside the body through a dialyzer, or "artificial kidney," to remove unwanted waste, toxins, and excess fluids. Most dialysis patients undergoing hemodialysis have a fistula as an access point, but that process takes some time before actual hemodialysis can begin. The subclavian catheter was faster and enabled me to undergo dialysis more quickly.

Once the catheter was in place, I was put on hemodialysis in the hospital and joined the ranks of some 520,000 Americans who must undergo kidney dialysis three times per week for about 3–5 hours, depending on the treatment schedule prescribed by the doctor. There are nearly 7,500 dialysis centers located throughout the United States, managed by the nearly 10 largest care providers, including Fresenius Medical Care of North America, DaVita Kidney Care, and U.S. Renal Care.

The DaVita center I ultimately decided on was about 15 minutes from my office. I arranged a schedule that would enable me to come to the center and undergo dialysis immediately following my workday. I showed up at the

36 It is worth noting here that multi-racial is not post-racial. Interestingly, many White supporters of the Obama campaign claimed the United States had become a post-racial nation. Although this was not true for the reasons they claimed it to be, it is true that skin tone bias appears to matter as much if not more than racial bias in mediating discrimination.

center at about 5:30 on Tuesdays and Thursdays, and earlier in the day on Saturday. This schedule required a fair amount of communication and negotiation with the DaVita kidney center staff because this was not a typical "chair time." Most evening patients showed up for treatment closer to 5:00 or 4:30. Of course, most patients were not working, and an allowance was made for me. My treatment lasted for 3 hours, and because the process of connecting and disconnecting to the dialyzer took some time, I did not leave the center on those weeknights until about 9:00 p.m. On a few rare occasions, the earlier inhabitant of my chair who was there for dialysis at an earlier shift was delayed in coming off of their chair. In those cases, I waited in the small outside waiting area until they were finished, and the unit was wiped down.

There were 15 units available in the center. Each day, almost all of them were occupied. The majority of them were located in a shared space that formed a large open circle. Patients in their chairs formed the outer part of the circle, with the nurses' station and equipment located inside the circle. Each chair had a small TV attached to its arm, and although patients were instructed to use their headphones, it was often the case that someone was not. The room hummed with the constant sound of mechanical beeps from the dialyzers, chair alarms going off, signaling the end of treatment and liberated TV sounds.

For each shift, there were a handful of technicians (they were not nurses) who were responsible for connecting and disconnecting patients to the dialyzer. Because hemodialysis involves the flow of a person's blood outside of their body, there was a well-established protocol to ensure the safety and well-being of the patients. That being said, the process was not without risks, and within the first two weeks of undergoing hemodialysis treatment, I witnessed an emergency that haunted me each time I sat down in a dialysis chair after that. The patient, a middle-aged African man, who happened to be seated in the unit next to mine, experienced an unexpected loss of blood pressure and collapsed. Paramedics were summoned and responded within minutes. They provided him with oxygen and swiftly took him to a hospital.

Most nights, dialysis for each of the patients proceeded relatively smoothly. During dialysis, I used the time to catch up on work-related tasks on my laptop and read. I did not enjoy watching TV on the tiny screen with a limited handful of channels.

What I watched more than anything else were the other patients. Sometimes I surreptitiously stole glances at the others in their chairs, and other times I brazenly stared, wondering about their lives and the circumstances that had brought them there. There were several patients who came during my chair time who were well acquainted with one another and could be seen chatting or joking at the beginning or end of their chair time. I was more curious about some than others. There was an older woman who tended to sit in the chair toward the back of the room. She wore a headcloth and looked very small and frail. I never heard a word from her. Across the room, in another chair, there was another woman, a middle-aged Black woman, who ended each dialysis treatment with a brief serenade to everyone in the center. Each night when her treatment ended, she sang the chorus to the song "Happy Trails" clear and loud.

Happy trails to you,
Until we meet again.
Happy trails to you,
Keep smiling until then.

On a few occasions, she wore a tiara. As a newcomer, I was smitten with her. The nurses and the other patients, obviously used to her, simply smiled or ignored her.

As I observed each of the other patients, I was struck by the fact that almost all of them were black or brown in skin tone. Whereas some of them were native-born, others hailed from other countries around the world and spoke languages other than English. Spanish was most prevalent, but Amharic could be heard among a few. What they (and we) all shared was the common characteristic of being people of color. Indeed, there were only two patients I saw during the entire time I underwent hemodialysis who appeared to be White. They stood out to me because they were White.

My observations aligned with the epidemiology of end-stage renal disease (ESRD). Minority populations in the United States have much higher rates of high blood pressure, diabetes, obesity, and heart disease, all of which increase the risk for ESRD.[37] African Americans are almost four times more likely than Whites, and Hispanics are about 1.3 times more likely than non-Hispanics to have kidney failure. As a brown-skinned African American, I fit right in.

As I considered this and thought about the challenge I knew existed in obtaining care, I was justifiably alarmed. If, as I hope to have shown here and in earlier sections, it is clear that people of color are diagnosed later and cared for in ways that are inferior to those of Whites, and if this particular disease afflicts more people of color than it does Whites, it is frightening to think about the predicament of the majority of ESRD patients. At what point

37 See The National Institutes of Health: National Institute of Diabetes and Digestive Kidney Diseases. Kidney Disease Statistics for the U.S. http://www.niddk.nih.gov.

are people being diagnosed? Is it possible that earlier intervention would have prevented them from reaching stage 4 and the ensuing need for dialysis?

Given the systemic barriers to health equity that others have written about and which I encountered personally, it is clear that the problem of the expanding number of patients requiring dialysis could be addressed by earlier intervention, more careful screening, and greater doctor—parent communication and trust, among other things.

Importantly, the treatment of kidney disease is a booming industry that generates huge volumes of capital for kidney dialysis providers. According to one report, the kidney dialysis market was valued at approximately $24.7 billion in 2018. This number is forecasted to grow to nearly $30 billion by the year 2023.[38] These numbers pertain to U.S. dialysis, and when one considers the global marketplace for kidney dialysis, these numbers balloon upward. The rising rate of kidney failure and chronic renal dysfunction around the world is expected to expand the market growth. According to the National Kidney Foundation, there are more than two million people around the world suffering from kidney failure who are undergoing dialysis treatment.[39] Thus, there are some very concrete reasons why the ESRD industry is growing.

Black and Brown people around the globe are contributing to the growth of the industry. Their overrepresentation within the ranks of those struggling with diabetes, obesity and high blood pressure ensures that they will be among the greatest numbers of people suffering from chronic kidney disease and requiring dialysis.

Discourse in public and private spaces around health equity has increased within the last year or so as a result of the COVID-19 pandemic. But many of these conversations have focused on access to care and the cost of care. Far less attention has been devoted to the underlying indicators of life quality that predispose members of minority communities to the environmental and economic stressors associated with obesity, diabetes, and high blood pressure.

Of course, these are not simple fixes but require a long-term commitment to addressing what is at the heart of much of these stressors—individual and institutional racism. I am referring to the negative sentiment that ultimately restricts people from accessing better jobs, neighborhoods, and schools. And of course, my problem was not a result of obesity, diabetes, or high blood pressure. It was the result of a failure to detect the presence of a rare disease

---

38 Yang, J. (2021). Kidney Dialysis Market Size in the U.S. in 2018 and 2023.

39 Grand View Research. (2017). Hemodialysis and Peritoneal Dialysis Market Size. http://www.grandviewresearch.com/industry-anlsysi/hemodialysis-peritneal-dialysis-marlet.

early on. Nevertheless, my experiences in trying to obtain treatment and care throughout this trial have made clear the challenges to access them. There are implicit biases, certain assumptions, and specific behaviors that when taken together are unwelcoming at worst and indifferent at best, and these affect patients of color most profoundly.

Chapter 5

BONE BIOPSY, STEM CELL HARVESTING, AND PRAYER

Multiple myeloma (MM) is an incurable blood cancer that occurs when malignant plasma cells grow uncontrollably in bone marrow. It is not curable, but doctors have made remarkable strides in treating it. As much as I wish that this never happened to me, I feel very fortunate that it did in a time when these pharmaceutical advances were possible. Whereas MM was a death sentence as recently as 10 years ago, it can be treated with a far greater life expectancy than was previously possible. AL amyloidosis is a rare disease that occurs when an abnormal protein, called amyloid, builds up in your organs and interferes with their normal function. MM and AL amyloidosis are similar diseases resulting from clonal proliferation and dysfunction of plasma cells and have likely outcomes in the kidneys because of protein deposits.

The[1] advances in the treatment of MM have been valuable for patients who suffer from AL amyloidosis.

In an earlier section of this book, I described the challenges of illness associated with a rare disease. Because fewer people are afflicted by rare diseases, they garner less research and investment from the pharmaceutical industry, which is driven by potential profits. Developing safe, disease-curing and life-saving medicines requires considerable time and money. According to the Tufts Center for the Study of Drug Development, the cost of developing medicine from invention to pharmacy shelves is $2.7 billion over an estimated 10 years.[2]

1 Suzuki, K. (2012). Diagnosis and Treatment of Multiple Myeloma and AL Amyloidosis with Focus on Improvement of Renal Lesion.

2 The Tufts Center for the Study of Drug Development is an independent, academic, non-profit research center at Tufts University in Boston, dedicated to researching drug development. It was established in 1976 by American physician Louis Lasagna. See the paper, Di Masai, J. A., Grabowski, H. G., & Hansen, R. W. (2016). Innovation in the Pharmaceutical Industry: New Estimates of R&D Costs.

The primary expense of developing any drug into something that consumers can safely use is the cost of conducting the research, including clinical trials, that will show it is safe and effective and ultimately able to secure regulatory approval. These expenses can range from $10 million to $2 billion, depending on what the drug is for. Importantly, it is not just the outright costs of the research that burden drug developers, but it is the loss sustained because a majority of drugs developed never make it to the market. According to one science writer, at least 90 percent of medicines that start being tested on people don't reach the market because they are unsafe or ineffective.[3] The $2.7 billion figure includes the cost not only of these failures but also of not putting the money spent on them into something that would give a more reliable return.

Treatment of those with rare diseases differs from treatment of those with more common diseases because of the low prevalence and lack of expertise in the case of rare diseases. Consequently, patients with rare diseases are forced to become knowledgeable about their own disease state in a way that patients with common diseases are not. Research has shown that, when compared to common diseases, patients with rare diseases are often more expert about their disease state than the doctors treating them. In these cases, it is especially important for the doctor to acknowledge the active role of the patient as an informed, involved, and interactive partner in the treatment process.

In the midst of this crisis and even through the inevitable "why me" phase of coming to terms with this new reality, I realized that I was extraordinarily fortunate to be living in the period when several life-saving therapeutics had been developed, proven safe, relatively effective, and were available to those with the means to obtain them (i.e., good insurance). I was also fortunate to have encountered Doctor S, who generally saw me as a partner throughout the process of treating me.

In the course of time, I soon came to see that the costs of the treatment protocol seemed to ensure that the drug developer would be generously compensated. It became somewhat routine for me to receive bills from the hospital totaling thousands and thousands of dollars. Receiving a bill for $89,000 that covered one day's treatment and a host of other accompanying charges was nothing unusual. These were all eventually reconciled with the insurance company, and apart from the initial deductible of $5,000, I was not required to pay additional fees out of my pocket. That said, I was very much aware of the extraordinary expenses this treatment entailed.

---

3 Herper, M. (2017). The Cost of Developing Drugs Is Insane. That Paper That Says Otherwise Is Insanely Bad.

There was also the matter of the monthly costs that I accrued that were associated with the dialysis treatment. Following nearly 3 months in two dialysis centers, which I visited three times a week, I had elected to pursue peritoneal dialysis (PD). Following the requisite training, which included 10 sessions with a PD nurse, a consultation with a surgeon and the insertion of a suprapubic catheter. The latter is a hollow, flexible tube that is used to drain urine from the bladder. It is inserted into the bladder through a cut in the stomach, a few inches below the navel (tummy button). This was done under a light general anesthetic. This enabled me to perform PD nightly in the comfort of my own home.

My kidney treatment included a brief monthly consultation with a nephrologist and a biweekly visit with the PD nurse, who took blood samples and provided me with continuing education about PD. However, PD is a patient-managed treatment and one that I did conscientiously every night. I was surprised to see the actual billing statement which the insurance company shared with me, indicating a daily charge of $3100. Each month, the kidney company billed them $31,000 for the suite of services they provided me, including the use of their equipment to perform the PD.

Some nine months into a prescribed treatment regimen that included regular chemotherapy and daily dialysis, the doctor who was treating me for the MM and amyloidosis, recommended a bone marrow biopsy. Although each of the biweekly chemotherapy sessions up to that point was preceded by a series of blood tests which provided important information about the chemistry of the blood, only a biopsy of the actual bone matter would provide definitive information about the efficacy of treatment. I agreed to this.

A bone marrow biopsy is performed on an outpatient basis and can take less than an hour. The bone marrow is the spongy tissue inside your bones that contains the red and white blood cells, platelets, fat, cartilage, and bone. In a biopsy, the doctor removes a small amount of the marrow from inside of the bone, and that sample is then evaluated in a pathology lab.

The biopsy for me was scheduled. This was during the height of the COVID-19 pandemic before vaccines were available, and the hospital was following strict protocols so that only patients were permitted in its facilities. Nevertheless, because of my anxiety about the procedure, the doctor made a special dispensation to allow my masked husband to be present with me during the procedure. The doctor performed the procedure in a small lab room in the infusion center. With my husband and a nurse present, she vigorously drilled into the bone on my right hip. Although I was provided a local anesthetic (lidocaine), the pain was excruciating. It was short-lived but extremely painful. Some 10 minutes in, the doctor stopped and ordered the nurse to provide me with an oral sedative. After waiting briefly for that to take effect,

Doctor S. obtained the necessary amount of cell tissue from the bone marrow. Sedated and exhausted, I slept nearly an hour before being gently awakened. My husband drove me home.

Two weeks later, I received encouraging news from Doctor S, who said that the results of the analysis revealed undetectable amounts of MM and amyloidosis, and that deep remission had been achieved. She explained that while this revealed success with the treatments, we would need to be vigilant in continuing to treat them. The protocol called for continuous monitoring along with monthly chemotherapy infusions.

Around this time, Doctor S also began talking to me about stem cell therapy. Stem cell therapy is a form of regenerative medicine in which the body's own stem cells and growth factors are used to repair tissue and replace diseased cells. Stem cells are the body's raw materials from which all other cells evolve. In stem cell transplants, stem cells replace cells damaged by chemotherapy or disease or serve as a way for the donor's immune system to fight some types of cancer and blood-related diseases, such as leukemia, lymphoma, neuroblastoma, and multiple myeloma.

Doctor S explained that by harvesting my healthy cells, I would have a ready supply for a stem cell transplant if I ever needed them. In this way, I came to think of this as a kind of insurance policy. Because I am generally a risk-averse person, I saw this as a highly rational strategy. I had no intention of ever needing to utilize these cells and undergoing what I knew would be an even more grueling experience of depositing the cells, but there was something reassuring about knowing that I would now have this option in the event that remission was shattered.

Stem cells have garnered a great deal of attention in the public eye because one source of stem cells which researchers have discovered is those that come from embryos that are three to five days old. Embryonic stem cells are obtained from early-stage embryos—a group of cells that forms when a woman's egg is fertilized with a man's sperm in an in vitro fertilization clinic. "Because human embryonic stem cells are extracted from human embryos, several questions and issues have been raised about the ethics of embryonic stem cell research."[4]

4 According to the Mayo Clinic. (2021). "The embryos being used in embryonic stem cell research come from eggs that were fertilized at in vitro fertilization clinics but never implanted in a woman's uterus. The stem cells are donated with informed consent from donors. The stem cells can live and grow in special solutions in test tubes or petri dishes in laboratories."

I was aware of the controversy surrounding the use of embryonic stem cells. But I also knew that adult stem cells was another option in the fight against this debilitating disease and it was in fact the only option for people diagnosed prior to the FDA's approval of the powerful drug Darzalex in 2015. I was equally as afraid as I was interested in stem cell therapy because of all that I had heard about it. I knew its effects to be grueling. I expressed my reservations to Doctor S.

Over the course of treatment, she continued to discuss the potential value of this approach for long-term maintenance. I thought more and more about it. During this time, I was feeling better and stronger, though I continued to be burdened by a cloud of uncertainty. How long would I have to maintain weekly infusion treatments? Would this have to be a routine feature for the duration of my life? Would I ever be eligible for kidney transplantation, given the indefinite course of this treatment? Answers to these questions weighed heavily in my decision-making, and I eventually began to see the value of harvesting my new healthy cells as a potential treatment in the future.

In retrospect, I can see that, however unconsciously, this became a new goal for me to set my sights on. Given the gravity of my sudden illness, I needed something to look toward. Deciding to undergo stem cell therapy was a huge undertaking. It gave me a goal and prompted my goal-oriented, achievement-motivated sensibilities. And, given the speed at which I was beset with not just one but two rare diseases that had compromised the use of a vital organ, I had not had sufficient time to adjust my identity so that it aligned with my now very vulnerable self.[5] I was struggling psychologically to maintain my sense of autonomy and optimism. All of these factors ultimately contributed to my willingness to undergo this first phase of stem cell therapy, that of harvesting my stem cells.

This turned out to be a very involved and complicated procedure that now required me to engage with another medical facility. I began a series

5 Not surprisingly, research has shown that when compared to the general population, people living with a rare disease and their caregivers report three times more often to be unhappy and depressed. These survey data show that patients with rare disease face a high burden and that healthcare to date does not adequately address the needs of patients with rare diseases. Moreover, even when compared to patients with cancer, those with rare diseases reported significantly higher unmet needs. In this study, 60 percent of patients with rare diseases did not feel sufficiently supported. See the study, Supportive care needs of patients with rare chronic diseases: multi-method, cross-sectional study by Depping, M. K., Uhlenbusch, N., Kodolitsch, Y. V., Klose, H. F. E., Mautner, V. F., & Löwe, B. (2021). Supportive Care Needs of Patients with Rare Chronic Diseases: Multi-Method, Cross-Sectional Study. https://link.springer.com/article/10.1186/s13023-020-01660-w.

of consultations with stem cell transplant specialists at the University of Maryland Medical Center. To be sure, my case was unusual in that I was requesting that my stem cells be harvested and stored indefinitely. While there was great enthusiasm for harvesting the cells and all of what that would entail, there was far less support for storing them. Indeed, this seemed to require quite a bit of back-and-forth deliberation among the staff at the University of Maryland Medical Center (UMD). Eventually, a decision was reached, and they agreed to store the cells indefinitely. In that moment, it appeared that kinder voices had prevailed. I learned later that insurance concerns had loomed large in the hospital's decision-making.

In addition to the cost-benefit analysis that played out, I was pretty certain that there was a corresponding lack of understanding on the part of the insurance company about why I was requesting that the hospital store the once-harvested cells. Because so much about the technical aspects of stem cells remains unknown, I was not surprised to learn that the decision to store the cells only followed after considerable negotiation.

Doctors' understanding about stem cells is still growing, and even as treatment with stem cells expands, much remains unknown. Although I realized this going in, I admit to being seduced by its potential. I knew that stem cells could be guided into becoming specific cells that could be used to regenerate and repair diseased or damaged tissues in people, and I was hopeful that if the disease returned, an infusion of my own stem cells might effectively overtake the cancer cells.

The preparation for the stem cell harvest began. This was a fairly involved process, and it included multiple consultations with the doctor and staff at the University of Maryland, online videos, a week's worth of self-injections, and one session of chemotherapy with Cytoxan. Cytoxan, an anti-cancer drug, is also used to suppress the immune system, and is usually given through a vein by injection or intravenous infusion. I received it as an IV infusion over the course of several hours. This one chemotherapy session proved to be particularly memorable because, unlike my ongoing treatments with Darzalax, this one treatment resulted in the complete loss of my hair. Although I was told that this was not likely to happen, all of my hair came out within three weeks of receiving the Cytoxan. More on this later.

One of the most common side effects of Cytoxan is nausea and vomiting. Because of this, the doctor provided me with a prescription for an anti-nausea medication. He said that I might experience nausea and that I should take these pills as soon as possible to alleviate it. I took the prescription to my local pharmacy and had it filled, but I did not take the medicine immediately following the infusion. I should have. I began vomiting uncontrollably. I would be nauseous for weeks.

Within days of the experience with the Cytoxan, I returned for a full day back at the hospital, during which time my stem cells were removed. The self-injections I had done in the preceding week stimulated the production of stem cells, which are typically found in small numbers in most adult tissues like bone marrow or fat. The challenge during the harvest was to obtain a sufficient number of stem cells. It was possible to fall short and so I had been prepared to return the following day for a second round. Laying relatively still for several hours, though not painful, was far from ideal, and I was hopeful that enough had been obtained on that first day.

I received the good news that evening that a sufficient volume of cells had been captured and would not require me to undergo the same procedure the following day. That was very good news. Although this was only half of the transplant process—we'd merely harvested my cells for later usage, I was physically drained and relieved.

Emotionally, I was pretty distraught. I felt incredibly weak and seemed to have permanently lost my appetite. When I looked in the mirror, I hardly recognized myself. And I received no follow-up inquiries or care instructions from the hospital. I had been dismissed following the procedure, and that was the last I had heard from the doctor or nurses who had managed my care at UMD.

Did they just assume that I would be fine? Once on this path, I could not resist the more sinister question: Did they care? That doctors routinely assume a certain degree of hardiness among Black patients relative to White patients is well established. Much has been said about this tendency and the downstream effects of it, which include delayed and incorrect diagnosis, inadequate treatment and failure to save the lives of Black patients. The healthcare industry and medical profession routinely fail African American citizens, and this has been written about most eloquently by historian of science John Hoberman in his book *Black & Blue* that provides a detailed analysis of the role of racism in medicine.[6]

It took about two months before I regained my strength and confidence in eating again. Yet, even then, something about this ordeal did not sit well with me as I was on the mend. How was it that I'd felt so miserable and suffered so greatly and had received no follow-up or inquiry from any of the doctors at UMD whatsoever? I was at a loss to understand. This was a heavy-duty procedure, as far as procedures go. How was it that no one had followed up with me?

6 See the book by Hoberman, J. (2012). *Black & Blue* for a detailed analysis and study of the origins and consequences of medical racism.

At the time, as I struggled to regain some sense of normalcy, I did not think much about this. It did not occur to me that I had been overlooked or that the doctor who was treating me had forgotten about me. Only some months later, after speaking candidly with Doctor S, did I come to terms with the apparent disregard and lack of follow-through from the doctors at the UMD medical center.

I could not help but wonder whether some lingering aspect of a "hardiness doctrine" had influenced the doctors' treatment of me. Had they fallen sway to the racialized thinking that permeated the medical establishment in the twentieth century? According to that dogma, Black people, who were fundamentally more primitive than Whites, possessed a natural immunity to disorders, to pain and to the diseases that more civilized humans, that is, Whites, suffered. This racialized way of thinking about African Americans served as a basis for the hardiness doctrine.[7] The latter conveniently justified White doctors' neglect and disregard for the population of poor Black people.

Contemporary investigations of healthcare inequity that have fueled conversations about the disparate treatment of people of color relative to Whites, that have uncovered disparities in diagnosis, treatment and mortality of patients and revealed the various ways that the medical establishment and healthcare industry routinely fail people of color, highlight the lasting effects of the hardiness doctrine. The obvious result of this false doctrine has been the tendency to overlook Black suffering and ailments. Indeed, one could rationally withhold treatment or concern from Black people because of their demonstrated superior physiology.

For me, this explained so much of what I was reading about and hearing about in the popular press. It may not have accounted for all of the examples of health disparities uncovered in the wake of the COVID-19 pandemic, but I was pretty certain it explained some of them. And, in my case, it helped me to understand how any one of the doctors responsible for my care had happened to overlook the importance of any follow-up with me.

In addition to the nausea that plagued me for weeks following the stem cell harvest and Cytoxan infusion, I noticed that my hair had begun falling out. Before undergoing the infusion, I had explicitly asked the nurse, a young White woman with a sunshine attitude, whether this would cause me to lose my hair. She assured me that it would not and that she had not heard of anyone who had lost their hair as a result of this. Because she said this, I was understandably alarmed when, two weeks after the procedure, I was nearly bald. I was completely unprepared for life as a woman without hair.

---

7 Hoberman, J. (2012). *Black & Blue.*

From a very young age, when I was a little girl, I valued my hair and envied that of others. Before maturity and well before hearing such adages as "a woman's hair is her crown and glory," I expended energy, time and thought on the hair that topped my head. Sometimes emulating another woman's hair, but always enabling a degree of satisfaction with my appearance. As a Black woman with a mixture of coarse and kinky hair, I was not unusual in the time and money I routinely spent on products, salons and accessories to beautify my hair.[8] Indeed, much like my complexion, my hair was very much a part of my identity. Whether it was long because of the addition of weaves or short and neatly trimmed, braided or loose, it was there.

I say all of this to underscore how traumatic the process of losing my hair proved to be. Had the doctor or nurse taken the time to tell me ahead of time that this was a likely, indeed possible outcome, the experience would not have been as bad. Not only hadn't they warned me about this, but when asked, the nurse assured me that this would not happen. It was extremely problematic.

As I noted in an earlier section, the state of disease I experienced as a result of the MM, amyloidosis and ESRD was accompanied by a noticeable change in my overall complexion. I was still struggling with this when I now confronted an entirely new challenge to my identity—that of complete hair loss. Now I really did not recognize the person who looked back at me in mirrors. This part of my identity was significantly altered.

Although it took me several weeks to pick myself up and move forward, I eventually did. When I shared the news of my now-complete hair loss with my very closest friends who knew about my health challenges, they all seemed to regard the matter of hair loss as relatively trivial. It was trivial in the grand scheme of things. That is, they concluded that if it came down to staying alive and losing one's hair, I had made the right choice. Only, from my perspective, it had actually come down to that. My decision to pursue the part of the stem cell treatment that included harvesting my adult stem cells was more "extra" than anything. It was not, at that point, a matter of saving my life. Nevertheless, I eventually came around to seeing it this way.

I went shopping for a wig and head coverings. From that point on, I greeted each day with a natural-looking wig. My co-workers, whom I continued to see and meet daily, never noticed that I now wore wigs. Of course, all of this took place conveniently at the very same time that people around the world who were able to, left their workplaces and began working from home.

8 See the article by Cheryl Thompson Black Women and Identity: What's hair got to do with it?

During this time, following the stem cell harvesting, I waited to hear of what my steps would be. The monthly infusion treatments had become more inconvenient than anything else, and I felt that I could reasonably manage them indefinitely. What I could not envision was a future that consisted of required daily dialysis. The prospect of facing life forever as a dialysis patient was overwhelming to me. I could not envision this, which is why I saw kidney transplantation as a desirable goal.

The UMD doctor who performed the stem cell harvest had advised me early on during our consultation that he would only be able to consider and recommend transplantation after having a window of at least two years' time of remission. The doctor, Doctor K, was not particularly sympathetic about this and maintained a fairly matter-of-fact disposition throughout our limited interactions. As a younger, White men, we did not connect across the gulf of our differences. He communicated his impressions to me, and I listened.

So, it was with this type of established interaction that he failed to follow up with me at any point after the stem cell harvest. I was not terribly surprised, but this compounded my already deflated sense of self. This was to be one of the lowest points of dealing with this illness that I experienced.

Not surprisingly, this would prove to be the beginning of an ongoing test of my faith. To be clear, I knew well that God was real. In principle, I also knew that life's challenges and crises tested faith. I knew that this crisis represented an opportunity for me to call upon and rely on God, ultimately strengthening my personal relationship with him. Whether my prayers would result in complete healing (i.e., it would be His choice), strength (i.e., I was not sure I could beat this disease), or peace (i.e., I was feeling terribly anxious), I knew that I needed to turn to God in a way that I had never had previously done.

I did my best to recite and recall specific scriptures that would not only strengthen and encourage me but also minimize the fear and anxiety that began to creep in. My fear ranged from whether I would be able to see my son graduate from college to whether I would ever look the same as I did before this illness grabbed a hold of me to what my husband would do without me. The most frequent phrase in the Bible is God's command to not fear, be afraid, or be anxious. I read and re-read many of those passages. In Isaiah 41:13, "For I am the Lord your God who takes hold of your right hand and says to you, Do not fear; I will help you." In Matthew 6:25, "Therefore I tell you, do not worry about your life, what you will eat or drink, or about your body, what you will wear. Is not life more than food, and the body more than clothes?" In 1 Peter 5:7, "Cast all your anxiety on him because he cares for you." In John 14:27, "Peace I leave with you; my peace I give you. I do not give to you as the world gives. Do not let your hearts be troubled and do not be afraid." In Philippians 4:6, "Do not be anxious about anything, but in every situation, by prayer and petition, with thanksgiving, present your requests to God." In Hebrews 13:6, "The Lord is my helper I will not be afraid. What can mere mortals do to me?" I reminded myself of some of the other many truths of His word like John 15:7: "If you remain in me and my words remain in you, ask whatever you wish, and it will be done for you."

Although I ultimately found peace in remembering these scriptures, I was at times slightly schizophrenic. I would be less than honest if I said that I wasn't angry with God. There were times when I resented him. I had pleaded and begged for my well-being, and that was not to be. Moreover, I realized early on that the process of obtaining care and medical treatment was itself an entirely separate challenge that would also require assistance from a higher power.

I did not avail myself of any of the existing support groups that I eventually learned existed for either of the orphan diseases I had succumbed to or the ESRD that challenged me daily. This was partly because of a lack of awareness and logistical convenience. One support group I learned about well into my treatment for amyloidosis met biweekly in a Zoom room. Although its organizer warmly welcomed all recipients of the email, I was not particularly enthusiastic about participating in the Zoom format with strangers to discuss the intensely personal experiences of disease battling and additional associated skirmishes. I remained in prayer and was grateful for the few people around me who knew of my predicament and earnestly prayed for me.

Truly, it can be seen that there is power in prayer, and research has increasingly sought to examine this claim of faithful believers. Indeed, as one author and physician writes in his book extolling the virtues of prayer in medicine, "faith is good medicine."[9] While this perspective is increasing, the faith factor in medicine is still treated somewhat skeptically by many in Western medicine who have observed inexplicable and miraculous patient recoveries but have responded to them with silence. This is somewhat at odds with a majority of Americans who believe in the healing power of prayer. For example, a 2000 *Time*/CNN poll found that 82 percent of Americans believe that prayer can cure serious illness, 73 percent believe that praying for others can cure illness, and 64 percent want their physicians to pray with them.[10] Ten years later, the Baylor Religion Study found that the most consistent predictor of healing prayer use among American adults was a reported loving relationship

9 See the book Proof of the Healing Power of Prayer (1998) by Dale A. Mathews with Connie Clark.

10 From the article by Ameling, A. (2000). Prayer: An Ancient Healing Practice Becomes New Again.

with God. Higher scores on this predictor were associated with more frequent healing prayer use.[11]

While there is no one agreed-upon perspective about the healing power of prayer or consistent evidence among the faithful that illnesses are reduced in severity or in any way lessened, there does exist an emerging empirical literature that is either focused on providing evidence of the impact of faith and prayer in the medical context and across multiple healthcare settings or debunking its usefulness altogether.

Consider a 2013 article appearing in the *British Journal of Nursing* that set out to explore the role of prayer in healing and its implications for nursing. To achieve this aim, the article provides a review of discourse and evidence on the power of prayer in healing. Ultimately, its authors conclude that although the evidence on the healing power of spirituality is inconclusive, there are indications that it has potential for the health and well-being of both patients and nurses.[12]

Another study, which examined the use of prayer among Australian women as part of the Australian Longitudinal Study on Women's Health, surveyed more than 9,000 women between the ages of 59 and 64. Results of the study revealed that a significant number of women used prayer and that prayer was significantly associated with health symptoms, chronic illnesses, and positive health-seeking behaviors.

There are, of course, critics of the notion of prayer for healing. Some of those who object are among the faithless, lacking any belief in a higher power or deity like God. Others, patients, doctors, and nurses, who are less adamant about this rejection nonetheless fall into this camp because of a simple failure to believe in what is not readily manifested and thereby witnessed in the medical setting or laboratory. As an example, in one study examining the impact of intercessory prayer on coronary care unit patients delivered in this study, intercessory prayer had no significant effect on medical outcomes after hospitalization in a coronary care unit.[13]

There is a wide variance in beliefs about the intercessory power of prayer. Not surprisingly, this kind of skepticism parallels even more pronounced disagreement about beliefs in God. I have found that talking about God or faith with

11 Levin, J. (2016). Prevalence and Religious Predictors of Healing Prayer Use in the USA: Findings from the Baylor Religion Survey.

12 See article by Narayanasamy, A., & Narayanasamy, M. (2013). The Healing Power of Prayer and its Implications for Nursing.

13 Aviles, J., Whelan, E., Hemkel, D. A., Williams, B. A., Kenny, K., O'Fallon, M., & Kopecky, S. L. (2001). Intercessory Prayer and Cardiovascular Disease Progression in a Coronary Care Unit Population: A Randomized Controlled Trial.

doctors and other healthcare providers results in one of two responses. Either they smile and nod their heads, or they freely acknowledge their own faith and beliefs. The latter has been far rarer than the former. Nevertheless, I had at least two experiences with healthcare technicians reflecting their own faithfulness.

At the first kidney center I attended, within the first few weeks of being treated for ESRD, I met a nurse who was assigned to my station. Nurse "Margaret" was from an African country. She was warm and, like the others there, sought to ensure I was being properly dialyzed. On one occasion, I was feeling particularly low and mentioned my concerns about missing out on something because I was there in the dialysis center. In response, Margaret asked me if it would be okay for her to pray with me. I agreed, and she began softly, though fervently, praying for me. She held my hands and closed her eyes as she asked God for healing for me. She prayed for several minutes, and at one point during this time, with my head bowed, I looked up and caught a glimpse of another nurse walking hurriedly past us. Though she said nothing, the look on her face reflected her disapproval. I do not know whether she disapproved of us publicly and visibly praying or whether she had particular issues with Nurse Margaret. Nonetheless, I found the diversion from the pragmatics and relative unpleasantness associated with dialyzing to be welcoming. I was then and remain grateful for Margaret's prayers.

One evening, some months later, following my transfer to another dialysis center, I had an unpleasant experience with painful involuntary skeletal muscle contractions (i.e., muscle cramping). During hemodialysis, patients can experience painful cramping. Although the underlying mechanism is not fully understood, a high ultrafiltration rate (removal of a large volume of water) and volume contraction have been indicated. It was my first time experiencing these spasms, and in addition to the pain, I was frightened and uncertain about what was happening to me. The technician assigned to me that evening, "Kai," rushed to my side, and along with the nurse, they both encouraged me to stretch and to calm down. Several of the other patients looked knowingly and sympathetically at me as I struggled. When the worst of the pain had passed and I had calmed down, Kai told me of a patient he knew of who had been miraculously cured. He told me that the patient had prayed and prayed and that he had consistently asked God for healing. And within time, he was healed.

I told Kai that I too was a "pray-er" and that I remained hopeful that I would be similarly blessed. To be honest, I don't believe that this is the way that things necessarily work, but I appreciated Kai's faith and thanked him for sharing this with me. I resumed my posture in the dialysis chair and endured the rest of the treatment time. When I was finally finished that evening, I was more relieved than I thought possible.

As I consider the faithfulness of Margaret and Kai, I note that, like many of the technicians and staff in dialysis, people of color were present. Indeed, one of the things that I noticed immediately in my interactions with the dialysis treatment industry was that many of the people directly engaged with the ESRD patients were people of color. Some of them were immigrants, and others were not. Whereas the doctors I saw treating other patients and those who treated me were either White or Indian, there was far more diversity among the actual technicians and nurses who oversaw and helped to perform the actual treatment for the patients. Did this really matter? On some level, I believe that it did.

In an entirely unfamiliar setting where I had little to no control and was trying to manage my success and survival in the face of the catastrophic loss of my kidneys, there was very little that was familiar. Communicating with others who looked like me helped.

It is well established that patients of color experience certain stressors with healthcare professionals because of their perceived differences.[14] In earlier sections of this book, I detailed an array of outcomes that have been identified across multiple studies, showing that the very fact of a difference between the provider and the patient accounts for disparities in treatment and care. When they differ from one another and the patient is a person of color, a member of a minority group, the normative tendency to generalize about minority groups (and other outgroups) leads providers to make assumptions about the patient that align with the provider's assumptions (i.e., stereotypes) about all members of that minority group. This means that the provider may discount certain factors or distinguishing features that would set that individual apart from the larger group to which they belong.

This bias toward homogenizing minority group people is manifested in an entirely different way when it comes to interactions between doctors and those whom they view as similar or as members of their own group. There is considerable research showing that most people treat members of their ingroup more favorably by recognizing individual differences that exist, giving them the benefit of the doubt in ambiguous situations and "going the extra mile."[15] In ordinary day-to-day interactions, this might result in minimal or benign differences in outcomes, but in healthcare settings where the

14 Miller & Peck. (2019). A Prospective Examination of Racial Microaggressions in the Medical Encounter.

15 Balsa, A. I., & McGuire, T. G. (2001). Statistical Discrimination in Health Care; and Balsa, A. I., McGuire, T. G., & Meredith, L. S. (2005). Testing for Statistical Discrimination in Health Care. *Health Services Research* 40: 227–252.

delivery of medical services can determine not only the quality of treatment and care but possibly whether a patient lives or dies, the impact of perceived differences looms large.

Of course, it is important to note that most doctors and other healthcare providers are caring people who want to help patients and do not consciously discriminate against any of them. However, the very nature of the medical setting, which emphasizes routine and economizes time, works against more meaningful doctor-patient interaction and communication. There is ample research showing that time and financial pressures force providers to engage patients in limited ways (i.e., based on their stereotypic beliefs), which in turn is driven by providers' biases about the patient's group.[16]

Woe to the patient of color who happens to be African American, is female and poor. The weight of these identities within a healthcare setting where most physicians are White (or foreign-born), male, and not poor is debilitating. There are so many ways that our healthcare system continues to fail them. This was the exact sentiment expressed by one of the women interviewed for Dayna Bowen's riveting text, *Just Medicine*. I include an excerpt of her remarks here:

> I think they just did not value African Americans. I think they have a stereotypical view of African Americans and they're keeping that. They're keeping that view, they don't want to let go of it. They feel that they are better in the world, or they just don't have any compassion. Or to me, they just don't care. They feel they are superior. Then on top of that I am in that poverty class. So, not only am I female and African American it's class too. I'm considered in the ranks of poverty using my Medicaid card. So, all three of these went against me when I went to the hospital.[17]

---

16 See e.g., Cooper, L. A., et al. (2012). The Association of Clinicians' Implicit Attitudes about Race with Medical Visit Communication and Patient Ratings of Interpersonal Care; Johnson, R. L. (2004). Patient Race/Ethnicity and Quality of Patient-Physician Communication during Medical Visits; and Cooper, L. A. (2003). Patient-Centered Communication, Ratings of Care, and Concordance of Patient and Physician Race.

17 From Matthew's, Dayna Bowen. (2015). Just Medicine. A Cure for Racial Inequality in American Health Care, 116–117.

Chapter 6

END GOAL—KIDNEY TRANSPLANT

Throughout everything that I have described so far, my end goal has been kidney transplantation. Without it, my survival depends on dialysis. And, while peritoneal dialysis provides a certain degree of control and convenience well beyond the burden of thrice weekly hemodialysis, it is by no means easy. It is only a substitute for a well-functioning kidney, and while it enables me to approach a sense of normalcy, I remain some distance from it. My ability to travel, to go swimming, or to even take a bath (I can only shower) is either impossible or extremely challenging now. And, of course, there are the many dietary restrictions by which I must abide.

The amyloidosis and multiple myeloma will continue to exist as simmering threats that will in the best-case scenario remain at undetectable levels. Whether this will require regular "maintenance" (i.e., infusion) remains to be seen, but the doctors treating this are confident about the current pharmaceutical cocktail's efficacy. They support and have encouraged me to pursue kidney transplantation.

In the United States, kidney transplantation was the first of the organ transplant procedures to be developed because of the availability of live donors and the critical technique of dialysis. In 1990, the American researcher and surgeon Joseph Murray received the Nobel Prize in Medicine for his pioneering work in kidney transplantation and the development of many new immunosuppressive agents, including drugs and monoclonal antibodies.

Since that time,[1] transplantation has become the treatment of choice for those with end-stage renal disease (ESRD), and at the same time, an understanding of the molecular and cellular events associated with the transplant has expanded considerably.

Today, kidney transplantation is a therapy for ESRD with benefits that go well beyond dialysis treatment. Kidney transplant not only provides a longer and better quality of life for ESRD patients, but it is also less expensive in the

---

1 Hamilton, D. Kidney Transplantation; A History. In Peter J. Morris and Stuart J. Knechtle. (2008). Kidney Transplantation 6th edition.

long run.[2] The current estimate for the complete cost of a kidney transplant is approximately $450,000. This includes physician fees, drugs, as well as hospital admission, procurement, and post-transplant costs, and while this fee of nearly half a million dollars seems expensive when one considers the accumulated costs for dialysis, it is clearly the less expensive option.[3] In my case, monthly peritoneal dialysis (PD) billing statements reflect an approximate cost of $31,000. In one year, PD costs were nearly $375,000. By year two, costs will have well exceeded what a transplant would have cost. Kidney transplantation represents a net savings in costs, both to the government and in total health care expenditures.[4]

In each of my interactions with the string of nephrologists assigned to me, I made clear my desire for a kidney transplant. With the exception of Dr. V (mentioned at an earlier point), all of the nephrologists have indicated their support and encouraged me to pursue this course of treatment. From the initial determination that dialysis would be necessary, a kidney transplant was presented as a viable option for me.

Unfortunately, the complexity of my illness has made transplant referrals more complicated. Upon learning of the amyloidosis and multiple myeloma, the kidney transplant specialists are less enthusiastic about this course of treatment. My oncologist referred me to a transplant team of specialists at the University of Maryland Medical Center. They recommended a two-year window of remission before considering a kidney transplant. It was during that window that I proceeded with the first stage of stem cell transplantation, in which stem cells are harvested.

At that time, the thinking was that these cells would be stored for future use should they become necessary. That is, if the MM and/or amyloidosis returned, we would proceed with the second stage of the stem cell transplant, depositing the healthy cells.

At nearly the end of the two-year window, I contacted Georgetown University Medical Center because of its reputation and track record for successful transplantation. This process involved an initial intake interview, a group presentation, and then a consultation with the lead surgeon on the team. When the time came to meet the surgeon for the consultation, I was

---

2 Garcia, G. G., Harden, P., & Chapman, J. (2012). The Global Role of Kidney Transplantation. *Kidney and Blood Pressure Research* 35: 299–304. https://doi.org/10.1159/000337044.

3 Michas, F. (2020). Average Amount Charged for a Kidney Transplant in the U.S. as of 2020, by category (in U.S. dollars).

4 Eggers, P. W. (1992). Comparison of Treatment Costs Between Dialysis and Transplantation.

excited as well as anxious. The consultation was conducted on Zoom, and the surgeon was a relatively young man of color. He did not have an accent, and in the two-dimensional space of Zoom, it was hard to determine his actual ethnicity. He was warm and personable, and he began the conversation very positively, explaining the hospital's desire to work with me. However, he was sorry to say that it would take some time because they would require me to complete a stem cell transplant. That would need to be done before I could be accepted for a kidney transplant. He assured me that no one would provide a kidney transplant to me in the absence of this step. Having a stem cell transplant was regarded as an assurance against the risk that the return of the MM and amyloidosis posed.

While I understood this in principle, I was crestfallen. Stem cell transplantation is grueling, requiring multiple pre-transplant procedures, a massive amount of chemotherapy resulting in complete hair loss, and a minimal two-week hospital stay. I had hoped to avoid this but came to understand that I would have to undergo it. I told the Georgetown surgeon I would do this, and he assured me they would be waiting for me.

Although I assured the surgeon that I would complete the stem cell transplant, I was far from enthusiastic about doing so. Nevertheless, this requirement provided me with a new goal. One that was pretty specific, closer in time, and attainable. This became my new goal, and I re-engaged the medical team at the University of Maryland to proceed with this next phase.

My last communication and contact with the people at UMD was nearly 9 months ago, when I left there under duress following the stem cell harvesting stage. I had experienced uncontrollable nausea and vomiting and had reached out to the nurse assigned to me. She advised me to return to the hospital, which I did promptly, driving myself the 50-minute route back to Baltimore. After asking me the same questions discussed on the phone, I was provided with an IV to counteract dehydration. I remained there for an hour, resting quietly in a private area of the infusion center. Following that, I was given a prescription for an anti-vomiting medicine and I returned home. I was nauseous for the next six weeks.

Because I never heard from any member of the UMD team again, and because so much time had passed, it was challenging for me to return to them. But I was desperate to be eligible for a kidney transplant. Dr. S., the oncologist with Washington MedStar, had communicated on several occasions with Dr. K of UMD. During one of those conversations, she shared with him my dissatisfaction, and she told him how I described my treatment and the lack of follow-up from his team. To his credit, Dr. K got right to the point when we met again for the first time, asking me what my recollection of events was. I described the agonizing discomfort I lived with being nauseous for nearly two months following the procedure, which impacted my ability to eat, the unexpected and complete loss of my hair and his failure to follow up with me at any point after the procedure. I was clear about my dissatisfaction and disappointment with their treatment and acknowledged returning only because I had to do so in order to proceed with a kidney transplant through Georgetown medical center.

I learned that this was all considered to be very unusual—from my complete hair loss to the almost constant nausea. What's more, I had inexplicably fallen through the proverbial cracks. He apologized and assured me that this would not happen again. We proceeded with the consultation for the second stage of the stem cell transplant.

Because of the tendency toward disparate treatment and the prevalence of disparities throughout the health care system, I was concerned about the extent to which stem cell transplantation was associated with such variables as patient race and socioeconomic status. My initial review of the existing literature was encouraging.[5] In one study, I saw that there were no observed differences between Black and White patients in the use of stem cell transplantation as a therapy for MM. Of course, this was only one study, which included 194 patients, but I found it encouraging.

Unfortunately, a more thorough review of the literature revealed a less sanguine picture and one that was consistent with the general trend toward disparate treatment of people of color throughout the healthcare system. In one analysis of the 2016 National Cancer Database for MM, the association between the utilization of stem cell transplant (SCT) as part of the initial therapy of MM and socio-demographic factors was studied, stratifying patients into mutually exclusive racial-ethnic subgroups. Results of the analysis revealed a significant disparity across racial groups for who gets stem cell transplant as a part of initial MM management and who does not, with those belonging to minority groups being less likely to receive this therapy.[6] There were a number of other studies resulting in similar types of findings.

---

5 See Lupak, O., Xiaoxia, H., Xie, P., Thanikachalam, K., Jabbour-Aida, H., Farhan, S., & Emole, J. (2021). Disparities in Utilization of Autologous Stem Cell Transplantation as Consolidative Therapy for Multiple Myeloma: A Single Institution Retrospective Review. *Clinical Lymphoma Myeloma and Leukemia* 21: 680–685. https://www.sciencedirect.com/science/article/abs/pii/S215226502100149.

6 There are multiple examples of research showing the existence of racial disparities in stem cell transplantation as a therapy for multiple myeloma. Some examples include: Ailawadh, S., et al. (2017). Factors Determining Utilization of Stem Cell Transplant (SCT) for Initial Therapy of Multiple Myeloma (MM) By Patient Race: Exploring Intra-Racial Healthcare Disparities; Shah, et al. (2018). Evaluating Factors Influencing

Taken together, this research attributes observed differences between Whites and people of color in the utilization of stem cell therapy for multiple myeloma to a combination of factors, including whether the medical facility was a research/academic one, patient insurance status, and physician bias, among other things. As an African American, I saw this as yet another way that I would need to actively work against the tide.

I knew that I would have to expend more energy like this, given my ultimate goal of kidney transplantation. It is well established that there are large differences between African Americans and Whites in overall kidney transplantation rates and in transplantation waiting times. Across all measures, Black patients suffering from ESRD and awaiting kidney transplantation fare worse than White, Asian American, or Native American ESRD beneficiaries.[7]

Results of one analysis exploring the time to transplant found that males were more likely to be transplanted than females, and at 1 year following renal failure, White persons were almost four times more likely to have received a transplant than black persons (22.7 percent and 6.0 percent, respectively).[8] According to the author of this analysis,

> The fact remains, however, that no matter what measure of transplant access is used, black beneficiaries fare worse than either white, Asian-American, or Native American beneficiaries. They are the least likely get on the national wait list, and have longer wait times once they do get wait listed. Consequently, their overall transplant rates lag far behind the other racial groups.

Not surprisingly, these differences also exist when comparisons are made for live kidney transplantations. That is, looking more narrowly at rates of live donor kidney transplantation (LDKT) across all major U.S. racial-ethnic

---

Receipt of Stem Cell Transplant and Time to Transplant at a Diverse Metropolitan Transplant Center: Do Racial Disparities Persist? Costa, L. J., Xing-Huang, J., & Hari, P. N. (2015). Disparities in Utilization of Autologous Hematopoietic Cell Transplantation for Treatment of Multiple Myeloma; Fiala Joseph, M. A., Finney, D., Stockerl-Goldstein, K. E., Tomasson, M. H., DiPersio, D. F., Vij, R., & Wildes, T. M. (2015). Re: Disparities in Utilization of Autologous Hematopoietic Cell Transplantation for Treatment of Multiple Myeloma.

7 See Eggers, P. W. (1995). Racial Differences in Access to Kidney Transplantation; Gaylin, D. S., Held, P. J., Port, F. K., et al. (1993). The Impact of Comorbid and Sociodemographic Factors on Access to Renal Transplantation.

8 Eggers (1995).

groups revealed lower rates for all people of color relative to Whites. Live kidney transplantation involves a living donor whom a recipient may or may not know who has agreed to provide a healthy kidney and live with one rather than two. These kidneys are preferred for transplantation because they are more viable. At the same time, they are more rare than those available from cadavers.

People of color in the United States are consistently less likely than Whites to undergo live kidney transplantation. Determinants of disparities in LDKT appear to operate on multiple levels, with some having to do with structural level factors and others at the individual level. Explanations for these differences include differences in socioeconomic status, chronic disease burden, healthcare access, and patient and provider attitudes, and knowledge about LDKT.[9,10]

What seems to matter most (apart from physical readiness) in decisions to transplant a kidney is the recipient's race and economic status (i.e., poor or not). In the United States, it is better to be White and it is better not to be poor across most sectors of society. However, in the case of organ transplant and kidney transplantation in particular, it really does matter. Studies consistently show that racial differences exist in access to referral, transplant evaluation, waitlisting and organ receipt, and even after adjusting for socioeconomic status, African Americans have a lower rate of transplantation than Whites.[11]

As evidence of this, consider the study provocatively titled "Access to Kidney Transplantation: Has the United States Eliminated Income and Racial Differences?"[12] The researchers analyzed transplantation lists and the census of 1,133 dialysis and transplant centers. Their findings indicated that White, male, young, nondiabetic, high-income patients treated in smaller

9 Purnell, T. S., Xu, P., Leca, N., & Hall, Y. N. (2013). Racial Differences in Determinants of Live Donor Kidney Transplantation in the United States.

10 See the website Donate Life American at https://www.donatelife.net/race-ethnicity-and-donation/ for detailed discussion about the way influences the likelihood of live donor kidney transplantation for people of color and African Americans in particular.

11 See as examples: Patzera, R. E., Perrymana, J. P., Schragerc, J. D., Pastana, S., Amarale, D. S., Gazmararian, J. A., Klein, B. M., Kutnerfand, B. N., & McClellan, W. M. (2011). The Role of Race and Poverty on Steps to Kidney Transplantation in the Southeastern United States; Hall, Y. N., Choi, A. I., Xu, P., O'Hare, A. M., & Chertow, G. M. Racial Ethnic Differences in Rates and Determinants of Deceased Donor Kidney Transplantation; and Patzer, R. E, Amaral, S., Wasse, H., Volkova, N., Kleinbaum, D., & McClellan, W. M. (2009). Neighborhood Poverty and Racial Disparities in Kidney Transplant Waitlisting.

12 Held, P. J., Pauly, M. V., & Bovbjer, R. R. (1988). Access to Kidney Transplantation. Has the United States Eliminated Income and Racial Differences? 4

units are more likely to receive a cadaver transplant under Medicare than are other kidney patients. While they did not compare rates of live to cadaver donations, their findings highlight the disparity in rates of transplantation for people of color, the elderly, the poor and women relative to men.

Nearly 20 years later, the data is similar. Another study found that race has an impact both waiting list entry and the receipt of a kidney transplant.[13] Taking stock of these findings for someone in my predicament can be discouraging. In addition to documenting a longer waiting time and a lower likelihood of referral to a kidney transplant, an analysis of the survey responses of physicians revealed their beliefs about Black patients' survival rates. They typically believed that there would be no improvements following renal transplant because co-morbidities, such as diabetes, hypertension, and obesity, are more prevalent in African Americans. These beliefs resulted in less overall support for transplantation among Black patients. Consequently, even after adjusting for socioeconomic factors, age, co-morbidities, and financial resources, Black Americans remained less likely to be listed for transplantation and continued to experience consistently longer waiting times.[14]

It is hard to convey the degree to which the decision to transplant is driven by physicians' beliefs and preferences, but it most certainly is. Physicians play a direct role in deciding whether to refer a patient for a transplant. When they wish to do so, they can share information with the patient, including anecdotes about success as well as in-depth accounts of the actual experiences of patients undergoing a transplant. In contrast, when they do not see a patient as a good fit for transplant, they can withhold information or fail to even mention it as an option. Whether direct or indirect, the physician plays a critical initial role in orienting the patient toward or away from a transplant.

Given the observed differences in diagnosis and treatment for White patients and people of color, and given the established reality of negative stereotypes and beliefs about Black patients relative to Whites, it is not surprising that racial differences in transplantation (across multiple kinds of transplants) exist.

---

13 Malek, S., Keys, B. J., Kumar, S., Milford, E., & Tullius, S. G. (2010). Racial and Ethnic Disparities in Kidney Transplantation.

14 See also for further discussion of the way patient preferences affect differential rates of transplant for Blacks and Whites. Patient preferences do not truly seem to be preferences but instead reflect physicians' preferences. Ayanian, J. Z., et al. (1999). The Effect of Patient Preferences on Racial Differences in Access to Renal Transplantation. *The New England Journal of Medicine* 341: 16667. This research showed that regardless of patient preferences, physicians were less likely to refer Black patients for transplants.

It is clear that racial disparities persist in waiting list placement and kidney transplantation. There are also observed differences in post-transplant treatment. Some investigators have documented differences in post-transplantation treatment, as evidenced by recent reports.[15] A post-transplant study of kidney recipients revealed that although transplantation dramatically improves patient-reported quality of life, some segments of the patient population, namely African Americans and women, do not benefit to the same extent as others.[16] The authors recommend that nurses recognize sociocultural differences in patients and how these differences affect care requirements.

Fairness and the Tyranny of Potential

Despite the aforementioned disparities that run throughout the entire American healthcare system, underlying today's healthcare system is the general notion, the idea, indeed the aspiration, that life-saving steps through clinical intervention must be taken. No matter the cost, the age of the patient or the likely duration of the prolonged life, current norms are to strive for therapies that will prolong life regardless of the quality of that life. "Clinical medicine materializes that potential in its therapies and in its discourse about therapies that offer, for ever-older individuals, additional months or years of life."[17] Thus, the potential of avoiding death through kidney transplantation is the backdrop against which much of the current kidney therapies are delivered.

Within the context of race and racial disparities, when physicians generally perceive patients of color to carry more risk than White patients, they are less willing to see them as viable transplant recipients and will be less likely to see or recommend transplant as a therapeutic option for patients with ESRD.

For kidney transplantation, the tension between this principle of potential routinely comes into conflict with principles of fairness about who is most deserving of a kidney. Kidneys remain extremely rare "commodities." There are far fewer kidneys available for donation than there are people who need them. People of all ages are in need of kidneys. Just as there is great variability in the ages of those in need, there are as many differences in the amount of

15 Fan, P. Y., Ashby, V. B., Fuller, D. S., et al. (2010). Access and Outcomes among Minority Transplant Patients, 1999–2008, with a focus on determinants of kidney graft survival.

16 Johnson, J. D., Wicks, M. N., Milstead, J., Hartwig, M., & Hathaway, D. K. (2007). Racial and Gender Differences in Quality of Life Following Kidney Transplantation.

17 From S. R. Kaufman's (2013) article p. 558, Fairness and the Tyranny of Potential in Kidney Transplantation.

time that potential recipients have been waiting, as well as the circumstances that account for their need.

Ethicists, anthropologists, and philosophers have devoted considerable attention to resolving the dilemma of deservingness in the kidney transplantation arena.[18] Among the issues considered, some are related to the safety of the operation for the donor, and others have to do with the identification of the recipient. While live donor transplantation eliminates the matter of fairness as it is directed to a specific recipient, other issues abound, including the potential high-risk status of the recipient.

In my own case, I was considered to be a high-risk patient because I am a Black woman who has experienced ESRD as a result of the unforgiving disease of amyloidosis/multiple myeloma. My initial conversation with the INOVA hospital system of northern Virginia resulted in a flat "no." following an initial telephone assessment with a transplant physician. I received a single-page notice in the mail that they would not be accepting me for consideration for a transplant because of the state of disease. This was in the first year of my diagnosis, and I was shattered.

Nearly a year and a half later, after experiencing remission, I reached out to Georgetown medical center. Following the evaluation, I was told that although they would be happy to work with me to secure and provide me with a transplant, they could only do so in good conscience with some reassurance that the cancer would not come back anytime soon. The only way to obtain that level of assurance was for me to undergo a stem cell transplant. Once I did this, I was assured I would be an excellent candidate for a kidney transplant. I underwent a stem cell transplantation in January of 2022, with the sole intention of being a good candidate for a kidney transplant.

Stem Cell Transplant and Beyond

The actual stem cell transplant took one hour on the day that I was admitted to the bone marrow treatment center of the University of Maryland Medical Center. The medical team was professional, courteous, and confident. I was optimistic and hopeful. My recovery in the hospital was supposed to include some period of time under two weeks before being released, after which I would have several weeks of recovery at home. As it happens, the medical

18 Mazaris, E., & Papalois, V. E. (2008). Ethical Issues in Living Donor Kidney Transplantation; O'Hara Jr., J. F., Bramstedt, K., Flechner, S., & Goldfarb, D. (2007). Ethical Issues Surrounding High-Risk Kidney Recipients: Implications for the Living Donor.

team was less skilled in handling my need for daily dialysis in addition to the standard protocol for stem cell recovery. There were complications that I experienced that reflected their inexperience with complicated cases such as my own. As a result, I was released prematurely two times from the hospital, only to be readmitted each time. I wound up staying in the BMT until for a total of three weeks.

I returned home incredibly weak, with a desire for nothing but sleep. I had no appetite and could barely walk the distance from my bed to the bathroom. I was in this state for about 10 days. I resumed work virtually. I continued to struggle with things like a lack of appetite, my desire to sleep, my speech being somewhat delayed from my thoughts, and my complexion having darkened so much as to be nearly unrecognizable. These were significant side effects that no one had warned me about.

What was most remarkable to me about the process of the stem cell transplant I underwent was the extent to which it affected my entire being. It not only impacted me physically but psychologically as well. What seemed like a simple injection process (of my own cells harvested nearly a year earlier) was actually a complex, highly invasive, and nearly overwhelming procedure. My words were slurred in the days following the 15-minute procedure, and it took some weeks for the fog that had settled just inside of my mind to clear.

I understand now that there are a number of lingering, bothersome symptoms that patients experience following a stem cell transplant, but at the time I did not know this. In one study exploring the first 100 days following a stem cell transplant, researchers used the symptom distress scale to identify the most frequently reported symptoms in a sample of 76 patients.[19] The most reported symptoms included fatigue, worry, and appetite change, which were the most prevalent.

Although my primary interest was securing a stem cell transplant to be eligible for a kidney transplant, in the days following the transplant, I could not entertain the thought of reengaging with the healthcare system. I was too weak and too raw, and the experience had been too much. It would take me nearly 6 months, along with prodding from my spouse, to reconnect with the Georgetown kidney transplant team.

During my recovery period, I was also required to get re-immunized for the host of vaccines I had acquired like most people in childhood and beyond. The process of stem cell transplant had wiped out all of the natural

19 Bevans, M. F., Mitchell, S. A., & Marden, S. (2008). The Symptom Experience in the First 100 Days Following Allogeneic Hematopoietic Stem Cell Transplantation (HSCT).

and acquired immunity I had before the transplant. From childhood vaccinations for chickenpox to the natural immunity I acquired from seasonal hay fever, to the ability to withstand the sulfuric outburst of onions, I was now extremely vulnerable. The timing of these vaccines, coupled with my now monthly maintenance chemotherapy, had to be spaced out carefully.

Six months following the stem cell transplant, with a few immunizations under my belt, I felt nearly normal and made the decision to reach out to Georgetown again. I was required to initiate the process of being evaluated again, given the time that had since passed and the change in my recent medical history.

It is impossible to overstate the significance of the recent advances in the treatment of light chain amyloidosis. I recognized how fortunate I was to be here now, not as recently as six or seven years prior, before the powerful drugs now routinely used for treatment were available. These advances had dramatically improved survival rates and several studies of long-term outcomes revealed that kidney transplants could be done successfully on those with amyloidosis who had undergone a stem cell transplant.[20]

Before the recent advances in chemotherapy, most patients receiving kidney transplants because of amyloidosis did not have long survival outcomes. Indeed, one study examining recipients of kidney transplants from 1973 to 1981 in 45 patients found the three-year survival of the patients with amyloidosis was statistically significantly inferior (51 percent) to that of the controls, those undergoing similar kidney transplants without amyloidosis.[21] More encouraging conclusions were drawn from another study in which all 46 amyloidosis patients were recipients of live kidney donations. In that study, the authors concluded that live-related donor kidney transplantation is a safe procedure for patients with amyloidosis.

This was good news to me and apparently well within the understanding of the Georgetown medical center transplant team, who, after careful review of my records, eventually notified me of acceptance into their transplant program. This is where I am today, undergoing the many tests required and waiting for a kidney.

20 Herrmann, S. M. S., et al. (2011). Long-Term Outcomes of Patients with Light Chain Amyloidosis (AL) after Renal Transplantation With or Without Stem Cell Transplantation.

21 See the study reported by Pasternack, A., Ahonen, J., & Kuhlbäck, B. (1986). Renal Transplantation in 45 Patients with Amyloidosis.

REFERENCES

Chapter 1 The Crisis of Diagnosis

1. Bryman, A. (2016). *Social research methods.* New York, NY: Oxford University Press.
2. Malinowski, B. (1944). *A scientific theory of culture and other essays.* Raleigh, NC: The University of North Carolina Press; and Franz Boas, F. (1924). Evolution or diffusion. *American Anthropologist, 26*(3), 340–344.
3. Khan, S. R. (2010). *Privilege: The making of an adolescent elite at St Paul's school.* Princeton, NJ: Princeton University Press.
4. Monti, D. J. (1992). On the risks and rewards of 'going native'. *Qualitative Sociology, 15*(3), 325–332. https://doi.org/10.1007/BF00990332
5. Wacquant, L. (2006). *Body & soul. Notebooks of an apprentice boxer.* New York, NY: Oxford University Press.
6. Goffman, E. (1967). *Interaction ritual: Essays on face-to-face behavior.* New York: Pantheon Books.
7. Wilkinson, C. A. (2017). Going 'backstage': Observant participation in research with young people. *Children's Geographies, 15*, 614–620.
8. Parkin, S. (2017). Observant participation with people who inject drugs in street-based settings: Reflections on a method used during applied ethnographic research. *Journal Addiction Research & Theory Volume, 25*, 39–47.
9. Alasuutari, P. (2010). The rise and relevance of qualitative research. *International Journal of Social Research Methodology, 13*(2), 139–55. https://doi.org/10.1080/13645570902966056. S2CID 143736805.
10. Smedley, B. D., Stith, A. Y., & Nelson, A. R. (Eds.), Committee on Understanding and Eliminating Racial and Ethnic Disparities in Health Care Institute of Medicine. (2002). *Unequal treatment: Confronting racial and ethnic disparities in health care.* ISBN: 0-309-15166-X.
11. Matthew, D. B. (2015). *Just medicine: A cure for racial inequality in American health care.* New York: New York University Press.
12. Hoberman, J. (2012). *Black and blue: The origins and consequences of medical racism.* California: University of California Press.
13. Marmot, M. (2015). *The health gap: The challenge of an unequal world.* New York: Bloomsbury Publishing Co.
14. Washington, H. (2006). *Medical apartheid: The dark history of medical experimentation on Black Americans from colonial times to the present.* New York: Harlem Moon Publishing.
15. Tweedy, D. (2016). *Black man in a white coat: A doctor's reflections on race and medicine.* New York: Picador Books.
16. Barr, D. (2019). *Health disparities in the United States: Social class, race, ethnicity, and the social determinants of health.* Baltimore, MD: Johns Hopkins University Press.

17. Ansell, D. (2019). *The death gap: How inequality kills.* Chicago, IL: University of Chicago Press.
18. Scheffler, R. M., & Arnold, D. (2017). Insurer market power lowers prices in numerous concentrated provider markets. *Health Affairs, 36*, 1539–1546.
19. Sommers, B. D., Gawande, A. A., & Baicker, K. (2017). Health insurance coverage and health—what the recent evidence tells us. *New England Journal of Medicine, 377*(6), 586–593.
20. Soni, A., Sabik, L. M., Simin, K., & Sommers, B. D. (2018). Change in insurance coverage among cancer patients under the affordable care act. *JAMA Oncology, 4*(1), 122–124. https://doi.org/10.1001/jamaoncol.2017.3176
21. Jemal, A., Lin, C. C., Davidoff, A. J., & Han, X. (2017). Changes in insurance coverage and stage at diagnosis among nonelderly patients with cancer after the affordable care act. *Journal of Clinical Oncology, 35*, 3906–3915.
22. McDavid, K., Tucker, T. C., Sloggett, A., & Coleman, M. P. (2003). Cancer survival in Kentucky and health insurance coverage. *JAMA Internal Medicine, 163*(18), 213–2144.
23. Salehi, A., Hashemi, N., Imanieh, M. H., & Saber, M. (2015). Chiropractic: Is it efficient in treatment of diseases? Review of systematic reviews. *International Journal Community Based Nursing and Midwifery, 3*(4), 244–254.
24. Caplan, L. S., May, D. S., & Richardson, L. C. (2000). Time to diagnosis and treatment of breast cancer: Results from the National Breast and Cervical Cancer Early Detection Program, 1991–1995. *American Journal of Public Health, 90*, 130–134.
25. Chang, S. W., Kerlikowske, K., Napoles-Springer, A., Posner, S. F., Sickles, E. A., & Perez-Stable, E. J. (1996). Racial differences in timeliness of follow-up after abnormal screening mammography. *Cancer, 78*, 1395–1402; and see Carey, P., & Gjerdingen, D. K. (1993). Follow-up of abnormal Papanicolaou smears among women of different races. *Journal of Family Practice, 37*, 583–587.
26. Schapira, M. M., McAuliffe, T. L., & Nattinger, A. B. (2000). Underutilization of mammography in older breast cancer survivors. *Medical Care, 38*, 281–289.
27. McCarthy, B. D., Yood, M. U., Boohaker, E. A., Ward, R. E., Rebner, M., & Johnson, C. C. (1996). Inadequate follow-up of abnormal mammograms. *American Journal of Preventative Medicine, 12*, 282–288.
28. Schieppati, A., Henter, J. I., Daina, E., & Aperia, A. (2008). Why rare diseases are an important medical and social issue. *The Lancet, 371*, 2039–2041.
29. Thomas, C. A. (1990). Re-assessing the orphan drug act. *23 Columbia Journal of Law and Social Problems, 413*, 435–436.
30. Landais, P., Messiaen, C., Rath, A., Le Mignot, L., Dufour, E., Ben Said, M., Jais, J. P., Toubiana, L., Baujat, G., Bourdon-Lanoy, E., Gérard-Blanluet, M., Bodemer, C., Salomon, R., Aymé, S., Le Merrer, M., & Verloes, A. (2010). CEMARA an information system for rare diseases. *Medinfo, 160*, 481–485.
31. Schiff, G. D. (2008). Minimizing diagnostic error: The importance of follow-up and feedback. *The American Journal of Medicine, 121*(5), S38–S42.
32. Schofield, P. E., Beeney, L. J., Thompson, J. F., Butow, P. N., Tattersall, M. H., & Dunn, S. M. (2001). Hearing the bad news of a cancer diagnosis: The Australian melanoma patient's perspective. *Annals of Oncology, 12*, 365–371.

Chapter 2 Black Women's Healthcare

1. IOM Report. (2003). Unequal treatment: Confronting racial and ethnic disparities in health care. https://nap.nationalacademies.org/login.php?record_id=12875&page=https%3A%2F%2Fnap.nationalacademies.org%2Fdownload%2F12875; IOM (2002).
2. Bailey, Z., Krieger, N., Agénor, M., Graves, J., Linos, N., & Bassett, M. T. (2017). Structural racism and health inequities in the USA: Evidence and interventions. *The Lancet, 389*(10077), 1453–1463. https://doi.org/10.1016/S0140-6736(17)30569-X
3. Feagin, J. R., & Vera, H. (2018). Future challenges: The sociology of racial and ethnic relations. In *Handbook of the sociology of racial and ethnic relations* (pp. 429–434). Part of the Handbooks of Sociology and Social Research book series. http://dx.doi.org/10.1007/978-3-319-76757-4_24
4. Black, L., & Stone, D. (2011). Expanding the definition of privilege: The concept of social privilege. *Journal of Multicultural Counseling and Development, 33*, 243–255. https://doi.org/10.1002/j.2161-1912.2005.tb00020.x
5. Hacker, A. (2003). *Two nations: Black and White, separate, hostile, unequal.* New York: Scribner.
6. Rothenberg, P. S. (Ed.). (2008). *White privilege.* New York: Worth Publishers.
   Branscombe, N. R., Schmitt, M. T., & Schiffhauer, K. (2006). Racial attitudes in response to thoughts of white privilege. *European Journal of Social Psychology, 37*, 203–215.
   Donnelly, D., Cook, K. J., Ausdale, D., & Foley, L. (2005). White privilege, color blindness, and services to battered women. *Violence against Women, 11*(1), 3–5.
   Blanchett, W. J. (2006). Disproportionate representation of African American students in special education: Acknowledging the role of white privilege and racism. *Educational Researcher, 35*(6), 24–28.
   Stone, J. (2002). Race and healthcare disparities: Overcoming vulnerability. *Theoretical Medicine and Bioethics, 23*, 499–518.
7. See for example https://www.washingtonpost.com/politics/poll-black-americans-outraged-by-george-floyds-death-but-optimistic-about-change-after-nationwide-protests/2020/06/24/1daad46a-b49e-11ea-a510-55bf26485c93_story.html. Retrieved May 31, 2021; And: https://www.npr.org/2021/04/13/986678488/grief-outrage-follow-another-police-killing-of-a-black-man. Retrieved May 31, 2021.
8. Sugrue, T. (2020). 2020 is not 1968: To understand today's protests, you must look further back. National Geographic, Race and Culture: published online https://www.nationalgeographic.com/history/article/2020-not-1968
9. American Heart Association. (2020). COVID-19 has unmasked significant health disparities in the U.S. Retrieved May 28, 2021, from https://www.sciencedaily.com/releases/2020/05/200504171856.htm
   Stark racial disparities persist in vaccinations, state-level CDC data shows. Retrieved May 28, 2021, from https://www.cnn.com/2021/05/20/health/racial-disparities-covid-19-vaccinations/index.html
   Racial disparities in Covid-19 case rates among young people were prevalent early in the pandemic, CDC study says. Retrieved May 28, 2021, from https://www.cnn.com/2021/03/10/health/disparities-covid-19-cases-cdc-study/index.html
10. Centers for Disease Control and Prevention. https://covid.cdc.gov/covid-data-tracker/

11. Golestaneha, L., Neugartena, J., Fishera, M., Billet, H., Gil, M. R., Johns, T., Yunesa, M., Mokrzyckia, M., Cocoa, M., Norris, K., Perez, H., Scott, S., Kim, R., & Belling, F. (2020). The association of race and COVID-19 mortality. *EClinicalMedicine*, *25*. https://doi.org/10.1016/j.eclinm.2020.100455
12. Selden, T. M., & Berdahl, T. (2020). COVID-19 and racial/ethnic disparities in health risk, employment, and household composition. *Health Affairs*, *39*, 8. https://doi.org/10.1377/hlthaff.2020.00897
13. Williams, D. R. (2008). Racial/ethnic variations in women's health: The social embeddedness of health. *American Journal of Public Health*, *98*, S38–S47.
14. Editorial. (2020). Henrietta lacks: Science must right a historical wrong. *Nature*, *585*, 7.
15. The Disparities in Healthcare for Black Women. Retrieved May 2020, from https://www.endofound.org/the-disparities-in-healthcare-for-black-women
16. Skloot, R. (2015). *The immortal life of Henrietta lacks*. New York: Crown Publishing Group.
17. Summerside, M. (2017). From Henrietta to HeLa: A history of racism and reality of distrust in the American medical system. *Gender and Ethnic Studies*, Honor's Archives. Retrieved May 2020, from https://www.colorado.edu/honorsjournal/archives/2017/gender-and-ethnic-studies-2017
18. Stern, A. M. (2005). Sterilized in the name of public health. Race, immigration, and reproductive control in modern California. *American Journal of Public Health*, *95*(7), 1128–1138.

    Ruteki, G. W. (2010). Forced sterilization of native Americans: Late twentieth century physician cooperation with national eugenic policies. The Center for Bioethics and Human Dignity. Retrieved May 2020, from https://cbhd.org/content/forced-sterilization-native-americans-late-twentieth-century-physician-cooperation-national-
19. Boggs, B., & Stone, O. (2013). For the public good: The shameful history of forced sterilization in the U.S. The New New South. Retrieved May 2020, from https://longreads.com/2014/11/19/for-the-public-good/
20. Centers for Disease Control and Prevention. (1995). Difference in maternal mortality among black and white women, United States (1990). *Morbidity and Mortality Weekly Report*, *44*, 6–14; Fang, J., Madhavan, S., & Alderman, M. H. (2000). Maternal mortality in New York City: Excess mortality of black women. *Journal of Urban Health*, *77*, 735–744.
21. Oparah, J. C., & Bonaparte, A. D. (2015). *Birthing justice: Black women, pregnancy and childbirth*. New York: Routledge.
22. The Black women's health imperative. 2020–2021 policy agenda. Retrieved May 2020, from https://3hqwxl1mqiah5r73r2q7zll1-wpengine.netdna-ssl.com/wp-content/uploads/2021/01/BWHI_NHPA_2020-21.pdf
23. Davis, D. A. (2018). Obstetric racism: The racial politics of pregnancy, labor, and birthing. *Medical Anthropology*, *38*(7), 560–573.
24. Davis, R., & Hilmantel, R. (2018). This is why we chose to talk about Black Women and infertility. Retrieved April 2020, from https://www.womenshealthmag.com/health/a23785945/black-women-infertility-letter-from-the-editors/
25. Popejoy, A. B., & Fullerton, S. M. (2016). Genomics is failing on diversity. *Nature*, *538*, 161–164. Retrieved May 22, 2021, from https://www.nature.com/news/genomics-is-failing-on-diversity-1.20759
26. Skloot, R. (2010). *The immortal life of Henrietta lacks*. New York: Crown Publishers.

27. Devine, P. (2001). Implicit prejudice and stereotyping: How automatic are they? Introduction to the special section. *Journal of Personality and Social Psychology, 81*(5), 757–759. https://doi.org/10.1037/0022-3514.81.5.757
28. Carbado, D., & Rock, P. (2016). What exposes African Americans to police violence. *Harvard Civil Rights – Civil Liberties Law Review, 51*, 160–187.
Brunson, R. K. (2007). "Police don't like black people": African American young men's accumulated police experiences. *Criminology & Public Policy, 6*, 71–101. https://doi.org/10.1111/j.1745-9133.2007.00423.x
29. Selmi, M. (2018). The paradox of implicit bias and a plea for a new narrative. *Arizona State Law Journal, 50*, 193–245.
30. Van Ryn, M., & Burke, J. (2000). The effect of patient race and socioeconomic status on physicians' perceptions of patients. *Social Science and Medicine, 50*, 813–828.
31. Greenwald, A. G., & Banaji, M. R. (1995). Implicit social cognition: Attitudes, self-esteem, and stereotypes. *Psychological Review, 102*(1), 4–27.
Blair, I. V., Steiner, J. F., & Havranek, E. P. (2011). Unconscious (implicit) bias and health disparities: Where do we go from here? *The Permanente Journal, 15*(2), 71–78.
32. Aboud, F. E., & Doyle, A.-B. (1996). Parental and peer influences on children's racial attitudes. *International Journal of Intercultural Relations, 20*, 371–383.
Barden, J., Maddux, W. W., Petty, R. E., & Brewer, M. B. (2004). Contextual moderation of racial bias: The impact of social roles on controlled and automatically activated attitudes. *Journal of Personality and Social Psychology, 87*(1), 5–22.
Snyder, M., Tanke, E. D., & Berscheid, E. (1977). Social perception and interpersonal behavior: On the self-fulfilling nature of social stereotypes. *Journal of Personality and Social Psychology, 35*(9), 656–666.
33. FitzGerald, C., & Hurst, S. (2017). Implicit bias in healthcare professionals: A systematic review. *BMC Medical Ethics, 18*, 19. https://doi.org/10.1186/s12910-017-0179-8
Dehon, E., Weiss, N., Jones, J., Faulconer, W., Hinton, E., & Sterling, S. (2017). Academic emergency medicine. A systematic review of the impact of physician implicit racial bias on clinical decision making. *Academic Emergency Medicine, 24*, 891–1036. https://doi.org/10.1111/acem.13214
34. Narayan, M. C. (2019). Addressing implicit bias in nursing: A review. *American Journal of Nursing, 119*(7), 36–43. https://doi.org/10.1097/01.NAJ.0000569340.27659.5a
35. Hall, W. J., Chapman, M. V., Lee, K. M., Merino, Y. M., Thomas, T. W., Payne, B. K., & Eng, E. (2015). Implicit racial/ethnic bias among health care professionals and its influence on health care outcomes: A systematic review. *American Journal of Public Health*, 105. https://doi.org/10.2105/AJPH.2015.302903
36. Epstein, A. M., Taylor, W. C., & Seage, G. R. (2004). Effects of patients' socioeconomic status and physicians' training and practice on patient-doctor communication. *The American Journal of Medicine, 78*, 101–106.
37. Ong, L. M., de Haes, J. C. J. M., Hoos, A. M., & Lammes, F. B. (1995). Doctor-patient communication: A review of the literature. *Social Science & Medicine, 40*(7), 903–918.
38. Bensing, J. (1991). Doctor-patient communication and the quality of care. *Social Science & Medicine, 32*, 1301–1310.
39. Matusitz, J., & Spear, J. (2014). Effective doctor–Patient communication: An updated examination. *Social Work in Public Health, 29*(3), 252–266. https://doi.org/10.1080/19371918.2013.776416
40. Buller, M. K., & Buller, D. B. (1987). Physicians' communication style and patient satisfaction. *Journal of Health and Social Behavior, 28*(4), 375–388.

41. Chandra, S., Mohammadnezhad, M., & Ward, P. (2018). Trust and communication in a doctor patient relationship: A literature review. *Journal of Healthcare Communications, 3*, 1–6.
42. National Academies of Science, Engineering and Medicine. (2002). Institute of medicine. Unequal treatment: What health care system administrators need to know about racial and ethnic disparities in healthcare. https://nap.nationalacademies.org/resource/10260/disparities_admin.pdf
    Also see NASEM. (2003). *Unequal treatment. Confronting racial and ethnic disparities in health care.* Washington, DC: NASEM Press.
43. Damon, T. (2015). *Black man in a White coat.* New York: Saint Martin's Press.
44. Street Jr., R. L., Gordon, H., & Haidet, P. (2007). Physicians' communication and perceptions of patients: Is it how they look, how they talk, or is it just the doctor? *Social Science & Medicine, 65*(3), 586–598.
45. Douglas, N. MD. (well + Good, 2020). https:///www.wellandgood.com/black-womane-health-care/

Chapter 3 Health Equity as a Perennial Pursuit

1. Montagu, A. (1942). *Man's most dangerous myth: The fallacy of race.* New York, NY: Columbia University Press.
   Gould, S. J. (1996). *The mismeasure of man.* New York, NY: W. W. Norton & Co.
2. Byrd, W. C. (2011). Conflating apples and oranges: Understanding modern forms of racism. *Sociology Compass, 5*, 1005–1007.
3. Sue, D. W., Capodilupo, C. M., Torino, G. C., Bucceri, J. M., Holder, A. M. B., Nadal, K. L., & Esquilin, M. (2007). Microaggressions in daily life. *American Psychologist, 62*, 271–286.
4. Mansoor, H. S. (2019). Modern racism but old-fashioned IIED: How incongruous injury standards deny "Thick skin" plaintiffs redress for racism and ethnoviolence. *Seton Hall Law Review, 50*(3), Article 8. https://scholarship.shu.edu/shlr/vol50/iss3/8
5. Katz, I. (1981). *Stigma: A social psychological analysis.* Hillsdale, NJ: Lawrence Erlbaum.
   Katz, I., & Hass, R. G. (1988). Racial ambivalence and American value conflict: Correlational and priming studies of dual cognitive structures. *Journal of Personality and Social Psychology, 55*, 893–905.
6. Delgado, R., Stefancic, J., & Harris, A. (2017). *Critical race theory (Third Edition): An introduction.* New York: New York University; George, J. (2021). A lesson in critical race theory. Retrieved from the American Bar Association August 4, 2021, https://www.americanbar.org/groups/crsj/publications/human_rights_magazine_home/civil-rights-reimagining-policing/a-lesson-on-critical-race-theory/
7. Simeonova, E. (2013). Doctors, patients and the racial mortality gap. *Journal of Health Economics, 32*(5), 895–908. https://doi.org/10.1016/j.jhealeco.2013.07.002.
   Ashton, C. M., Haidet, P., Paterniti, D. A., Collins, T. C., Gordon, H. S., O'Malley, K., Petersen, L. A., Sharf, B. F., Suarez-Almazor, M. E., Wray, N. P., & Street Jr., R. L. (2003, February). Racial and ethnic disparities in the use of health services. Bias, preferences, or poor communication? *General Internal Medicine, 18*, 146–152.
   Cooper-Patrick, L., Gallo, J. J., Gonzales, J. J., Vu, H. T., Powe, N. R., Nelson, C., & Ford, D. E. (1999). Race, gender, and partnership in the patient-physician relationship. *Journal of American Medical Association, 282*(6), 583–589. https://doi.org/10.1001/jama.282.6.583.

Bleich, S. N., Simon, A. E., & Cooper, L. A. (2012). Impact of patient–Doctor race concordance on rates of weight-related counseling in visits by black and white obese individuals. *Obesity*, *20*(3), 562–570.

8. LaVeist, T. A., & Nuru-Jeter, A. (2002). Is doctor-patient race concordance associated with greater satisfaction with care? *Journal of Health & Social Behavior*, *43*(3), 296–306.
9. Klonoff, E. A. (2009). Disparities in the provision of medical care: An outcome in search of an explanation. *Journal of Behavioral Medicine*, *32*. https://doi.org/10.1007/s10865-008-9192-1
10. Smedley, B. D., Stith, A. Y., & Nelson, A. R. (2003). Editors, committee on understanding and eliminating racial and ethnic disparities in health care unequal treatment: Confronting racial and ethnic disparities in health care. ISBN: 0-309-15166-X. This PDF is available from the National Academies Press at http://www.nap.edu/catalog/12875.html
11. Bikbov, B., et al. (2020). Global, regional, and national burden of chronic kidney disease, 1990–2017: A systematic analysis for the Global Burden of Disease Study 2017. *The Lancet*, *395*, 709–733.
12. Liyanage, T., et al. (2015). Worldwide access to treatment for end-stage kidney disease: A systematic review. *The Lancet*, *385*, 1975–1982.
13. Himmelfarb, J., Vanholder, R., Mehrotra, R., et al. (2020). The current and future landscape of dialysis. *National Review of Nephrology*, *16*, 573–585. https://doi.org/10.1038/s41581-020-0315-4
14. Consumer Reports. (2022). Where to get free Medicare advice? https://www.consumerreports.org/cro/2014/10/where-to-get-free-medicare-advice/index.htm
15. LaRosa, J. (2019). U.S. kidney dialysis clinics form a profitable $24 billion industry. Retrieved January 8, 2021, from https://blog.marketresearch.com/u.s.-kidney-dialysis-clinics-form-a-profitable-24-billion-industry
16. Eneanya, N. D., Yang, W., & Reese, P. P. (2019). Reconsidering the consequences of using race to estimate kidney function. *Journal of American Medical Association*, *322*, 113–114.
17. Kuzawa, C. W., & Elizabeth Sweet, E. (2008). Epigenetics and the embodiment of race: Developmental origins of US racial disparities in cardiovascular health. *American Journal of Human Biology*, *21*, 2–15. https://doi.org/10.1002/ajhb.20822
    Vick, A. D., & Burris, H. H. (2017). Epigenetics and health disparities. *Current Epidemiology Reports*, *4*, 31–37.
18. Vyas, D. A., Eisenstein, L. G., & Jones, D. S. (2020). Hidden in plain sight – Reconsidering the use of race correction in clinical algorithm. *The New England Journal of Medicine*, *383*, 9. Retrieved August 9, 2021, from https://www.nejm.org/doi/pdf/10.1056/NEJMms2004740
19. Hallab, A., & Wish, J. B. (2018). Employment among patients on dialysis. An unfulfilled promise. *Clinical Journal of the American Society for Nephrology*, *13*(2), 203–204. Published online January 18, 2018. https://doi.org/10.2215/CJN.13491217
20. Kutner, N., Bowles, T., Zhang, R., Huang, Y., & Pastan, S. (2008). Dialysis facility characteristics and variation in employment rates: A national study. *Clinical Journal of the American Society for Nephrology*, *3*(1), 111–116.
21. National Kidney Foundation. Retrieved August 11, 2021, from https://www.kidney.org/atoz/content/peritoneal

22. Centers for Disease Control and Prevention. Retrieved August 12, 2021, from https://www.cdc.gov/vaccines/covid-19/planning/dialysis-partners-jurisdictions.html

Chapter 4 The Subtlety of Skin Tone Bias and Racism in Access to Quality Care

1. Wilson, M., Russell, K., & Hall, R. (2013). *The color complex: The politics of skin color in a new millennium.* New York: Knopf Doubleday Publishing Group.
2. Hunter, M. (2007). The persistent problem of colorism: Skin tone, status, and inequality. *Sociology Compass, 1*(1), 237–254. https://doi.org/10.1111/j.1751-9020.2007.00006.x
3. Hodes, M. (1997). *White women, Black men: Illicit sex in the nineteenth-century south.* New Haven: Yale University Press.
4. Herring, C., Keith, V. M., & Horton, H. D. (Eds.). (2003). *Skin deep: Race and complexion in the color-blind era.* Chicago, IL: University of Illinois Press.
5. Wirth, L., & Goldhamer, H. (1944). *Characteristics of the American Negro.* New York/London: Harper & Brothers Publishers.
   Frazier, E. F. (1957). *Black bourgeoisie.* Glencoe, Illinois: Free Press.
6. Wilson, M., Russell, K., & Hall, R. (2013). *The color complex: The politics of skin color in a new millennium.* New York: Knopf Doubleday Publishing Group.
7. Monk, E. P. (2021). The unceasing significance of colorism: Skin tone stratification in the United States. Daedalus: American Academy of Arts & Sciences. Retrieved August 28, 2021, from https://www.amacad.org/publication/colorism-skin-tone-stratification-united-states
   Jordan, W. (1968). *White over Black.* Chapel Hill, NC: University of North Carolina Press.
8. Rondilla, J., & Spickard, P. (2007). *Is lighter better?* Lanham, MD: Rowman & Littlefield.
9. Jones, V. (2004). Pride or prejudice? A formally taboo topic among Asian-Americans and Latinos comes out into the open as skin tone consciousness sparks a Backlash. *Boston Globe*, August 19, 2004.
10. Hunter, M. (2007). The persistent problem of colorism: Skin tone, status, and inequality. *Sociology Compass, 1*(1), 237–254.
11. Maddox, K. B. (2004). Perspectives on racial Phenotypicality bias. *Personality and Social Psychology Review, 8*(4), 383–401.
12. Goldsmith, A. H., Hamilton, D., & Darity, W. Jr. (2007). From dark to light: Skin color and Wages among African-Americans. *The Journal of Human Resources, 42*(4), 701–738.
13. Monk, E. P. (2014). Skin tone stratification among Black Americans, 2001–2003. *Social Forces, 92*(4), 1313–1337.
14. Norwood, K. J. (2014). *Color matters.* New York: Routledge.
15. Maddox, K., & Gray, S. A. (2002). Cognitive representations of Black Americans: Reexploring the role of skin tone. *Personality and Social Psychology Bulletin, 28*(2), 250–259. https://doi.org/10.1177/0146167202282010
    Hagiwara, N., Kash, D. A., & Cesario, J. (2012). The independent effects of skin tone and facial features on Whites' affective reactions to Blacks. *Journal of Experimental Social Psychology, 48*(4), 892–898.

16. Donovan, R. A. (2011). Tough or tender: (Dis)similarities in White college students' perceptions of Black and White women. *Psychology of Women Quarterly*, *35*, 458–468. https://doi.org/10.1177/0361684311406874
17. Lemons, J. S. (1977). Black stereotypes as reflected in popular culture, 1880–1920. *American Quarterly*, *29*(1), 102–116.
18. Drake, S. C., & Cayton, H. R. (1962). *Black metropolis*. New York: Harper and Row.
    Freeman, H. E., Armor, D., Ross, J. M., & Pettigrew, T. F. (1966). Color gradation and attitudes among middle-income negroes. *American Sociological Review*, *31*, 365–375.
    Powell-Hopson, D., & Hopson, D. S. (1988). Implications of doll color preferences among black preschool children and white preschool children. *The Journal of Black Psychology*, *14*, 57–63.
    Edward, R. H. (1970). Skin color, life chances, and anti-white attitudes. *Social Problems*, *18*, 164–179.
19. Terkildsen, N. (1993). When White voters evaluate black candidates: The processing implications of candidate skin color, prejudice, and self-monitoring. *American Journal of Political Science*, *37*, 1032–1053.
    Caliendo, S. M., & Mcilwain, C. D. (2006). Minority candidates, media framing, and racial cues in the 2004 election. *The Harvard International Journal of Press/Politics*, *11*, 45–69.
20. Blair, I. V., Judd, C. M., & Chapleau, K. M. (2004). The influence of Afrocentric facial features in criminal sentencing. *Psychological Science*, *15*, 674–679.
    Eberhardt, J. L., Goff, P. A., Purdie, V. J., & Davies, P. G. (2004). Seeing Black: Race, crime, and visual processing. *Journal of Personality and Social Psychology*, *87*, 876–893. https://doi.org/10.1037/0022-3514.87.6.876
21. Viglione, J., Hannon, L., & DeFina, R. (2011). The impact of light skin on prison time for black female offenders. *The Social Science Journal*, *48*(1), 250–258. https://doi.org/10.1016/j.soscij.2010.08.003
22. Hughes, B., & Hertel, M. (1990). The significance of color remains: A study of life chances, mate selection, and ethnic consciousness among Black Americans. *Social Forces*, *68*, 1105–1120.
23. Russell, K., Wilson, M., & Hall, R. (1992). *The color complex*. New York: Doubleday.
24. Hunter, M. (2005). *Race, gender, and the politics of skin tone*. New York: Routledge.
25. Gomez, C. (2000). The continual significance of skin color: An exploratory study of Latinos in the northeast. *Hispanic Journal of Behavioral Sciences*, *22*, 94–103.
    Hughes, B., & Hertel, M. (1990). The significance of color remains: A study of life chances, mate selection, and ethnic consciousness among Black Americans. *Social Forces*, *68*, 1105–1120.
    Hunter, M. (2002). If you're light, you're alright: Light skin color as social capital for women of color. *Gender & Society*, *16*, 175–193.
26. Fears, D. (2003). Race divides hispanics, report says; integration and income vary with skin color. *Washington Post*, July 14, 2003.
27. Rodolfo, E., & Franz, M. (2002). Latino phenotypic discrimination revisited: The impact of skin color on occupational status. *Social Science Quarterly*, *83*, 612–623.
28. Hunter, M. (2005). *Race, gender, and the politics of skin tone*. New York: Routledge.
29. Hunter, M. (2005). *Race, gender, and the politics of skin tone*. New York: Routledge.
30. Ellis, P. M. (2021). The unceasing significance of colorism: Skin tone stratification in the United States. *Daedalus*, *150*(2), 76–90.

31. Laidley, T., Domingue, B., & Sinsub, P., et al. (2019). New evidence of skin color bias and health outcomes using sibling difference models: A research note. *Demography*, *56*(2), 753–762.
32. Laidley, T., Domingue, B., Sinsub, P., Mullan Harris, K., & Conley, D. (2019). New evidence of skin color bias and health outcomes using sibling difference models: A research note. *Demography*, *56*, 753–762. https://doi.org/10.1007/s13524-018-0756-6
33. Bowleg, Lisa. (2012). The Problem With the Phrase Women and Minorities: Intersectionality—an Important Theoretical Framework for Public Health. Accepted: February 20, 2012. Published Online: June 07, 2012. https://ajph.aphapublications.org/doi/10.2105/AJPH.2012.300750.
34. Workman, K. (2021). Using an intersectionality framework to examine disparities in the steps to kidney transplantation in patients with end stage renal disease. University of Richmond, Honors Thesis. https://scholarship.richmond.edu/cgi/viewcontent.cgi?article=2574&context=honors-theses
35. Slaughter-Acey, J. C., Sneed, D., Parker, L., & Keith, V. M. (2019). Skin tone matters: Racial microaggressions and delayed prenatal care. *American Journal of Preventive Medicine*, *57*, 321–329.
36. Craig-Henderson, Kellina M. (2014). Colorism and interracial intimacy: How skin color matters. In Kimberly Jade Norwood (Ed.), *Color matters: Skin tone bias and the myth of a postracial America*. New York, NY: Routledge. https://aadl.org/catalog/record/10054646.
37. The National Institutes of Health: National Institute of Diabetes and Digestive Kidney Diseases. Kidney Disease Statistics for the U.S. http:www.niddk.nih.gov.
38. Yang, J. (2022). Kidney dialysis market size in the U.S. in 2018 and 2023. Statista Research Development. https://www.statista.com/statistics/1110120/us-kidney-dialysis-market-valuation/
39. Grand View Research. (2017). Hemodialysis and peritoneal dialysis market size. http://www.grandviewresearch.com/industry-anlsysi/hemodialysis-peritneal-dialysis-marlet

Chapter 5 Bone Biopsy, Stem Cell Harvesting and Prayer

1. Suzuki, K. (2012). Diagnosis and treatment of multiple myeloma and AL amyloidosis with focus on improvement of renal lesion. *Clinical and Experimental Nephrology*, *16*(5), 659–671. https://doi.org/10.1007/s10157-012-0684-5
2. Di Masai, J. A., Grabowski, H. G., & Hansen, R. W. (2016). Innovation in the pharmaceutical industry: New estimates of R&D costs. *Journal of Health Economics*, *47*, 20–33.
3. Herper, M. (2017). The cost of developing drugs is insane. That paper that says otherwise is insanely bad. *Forbes*. Retrieved October 29, 2017, from https://www.forbes.com/sites/matthewherper/2017/10/16/the-cost-of-developing-drugs-is-insane-a-paper-that-argued-otherwise-was-insanely-bad/?sh=5b4f054b2d45
4. Mayo Clinic. Retrieved October 22, 2021, from https://www.mayoclinic.org/tests-procedures/bone-marrow-transplant/in-depth/stem-cells/art-20048117
5. Depping, M. K., Uhlenbusch, N., Kodolitsch, Y. V., Klose, H. F. E., Mautner, V. F., & Löwe, B. (2021). Supportive care needs of patients with rare chronic diseases: Multi-method, cross-sectional study. *Orphanet Journal of Rare Diseases*, *16*(44). Retrieved October 29, 2021, from https://link.springer.com/article/10.1186/s13023-020-01660-w
6. Hoberman, J. (2012). *Black & blue*. California: University of California Press.

7. Hoberman, J. (2012). *Black & blue.* California: University of California Press.
8. Thompson, C. (2008-2009). Black women and identity: What's hair got to do with it? *Michigan Feminist Studies, 22*(1). Issue title: Politics and Performativity. http://hdl.handle.net/2027/spo.ark5583.0022.105
9. Matthews, D. A. (1998). *Proof of the healing power of prayer.* New York: Penguin Books.
10. Ameling, A. (2000). Prayer: An ancient healing practice becomes new again. *Holistic Health and Nursing Practice, 14*(3), 40–48. Retrieved May 11, 2021, from https://journals.lww.com/hnpjournal/Abstract/2000/04000/Prayer__An_Ancient_Healing_Practice_Becomes_New.8.aspx
11. Levin, J. (2016). Prevalence and religious predictors of healing prayer use in the USA: Findings from the Baylor religion survey. *Journal of Religion and Health, 55,* 1136–1158.
12. See Narayanasamy, A., & Narayanasamy, M. (2013). The healing power or prayer and its implications for nursing. *British Journal of Nursing, 17*(6). Retrieved September 27, 2013, from https://doi.org/10.12968/bjon.2008.17.6.28907
13. Aviles, J., Whelan, E., Hemkel, D. A., Williams, B. A., Kenny, K., O'Fallon, M., & Kopecky, S. L. (2001). Intercessory prayer and cardiovascular disease progression in a coronary care unit population: A randomized controlled trial. *Mayo Clinic Proceedings, 76,* 1192–1198.
14. Miller, L. R., & Peck, B. M. (2019). A prospective examination of racial microaggressions in the medical encounter. *Journal of Racial and Ethnic Health Disparities, 7,* 519–527.
15. Balsa, A. I., & McGuire, T. G. (2001). Statistical discrimination in Health Care. *Journal of Health Economics, 20*(6), 881–907. https://doi.org/10.1016/s0167-6296(01)00101-1

    Balsa, A. I., McGuire, T. G., & Meredith, L. S. (2005). Testing for statistical discrimination in health care. *Health Services Research, 40,* 227–252.
16. Cooper, L. A., et al. (2012). The association of clinicians' implicit attitudes about race with medical visit communication and patient ratings of interpersonal care. *American Journal of Public Health, 102,* 979–987.

    Johnson, R. L. (2004). Patient race/ethnicity and quality of patient-physician communication during medical visits. *American Journal of Public Health, 94,* 2084–2090.

    Cooper, L. A. (2003). Patient-centered communication, ratings of care, and concordance of patient and physician race. *Annals of Internal Medicine, 139,* 907–915.
17. Matthew, D. B. (2015). *Just medicine. A cure for racial inequality in American health care.* New York: New York University Press.

Chapter 6 End Goal –Kidney Transplant

1. Hamilton, D. (2008). Kidney transplantation; a history. In P. J. Morris & S. J. Knechtle (Eds.), *Kidney transplantation* (6th ed., pp. 1–9). Philadelphia, PA: Saunders Elsevier.
2. Garcia, G. G., Harden, P., & Chapman, J. (2012). The global role of kidney transplantation. *Kidney and Blood Pressure Research, 35,* 299–304. https://doi.org/10.1159/000337044
3. Michas, F. (2020). Average amount charged for a kidney transplant in the U.S. as of 2020, by category (in U.S. dollars). *Statista.* https://www.statista.com/statistics/1100710/organ-transplantation-costs-breakdown-us/

4. Eggers, P. W. (1992). Comparison of treatment costs between dialysis and transplantation. *Seminars in Nephrology, 12*(3), 284–289.
5. Lupak, O., Xiaoxia, H., Xie, P., Thanikachalam, K., Jabbour-Aida, H., Farhan, S., & Emole, J. (2021). Disparities in utilization of autologous stem cell transplantation as consolidative therapy for multiple myeloma: A single institution retrospective review. *Clinical Lymphoma Myeloma and Leukemia, 21*, 680–685. https://www.sciencedirect.com/science/article/abs/pii/S215226502100149
6. Ailawadh, S., et al. (2017). Factors determining utilization of Stem Cell Transplant (SCT) for initial therapy of Multiple Myeloma (MM) by patient race: Exploring intra-racial healthcare disparities. *Blood, 130*(Supplement 1), 860. https://doi.org/10.1182/blood.V130.Suppl_1.860.860
   Shah, H., Kim, S., Klimecki, S., Uberti, J. P., Schiffer, C. A., & Seymour, E. K. (2018). Evaluating factors influencing receipt of stem cell transplant and time to transplant at a diverse metropolitan transplant center: Do racial disparities persist? *Blood, 132*(Supplement 1), 323. http://doi.org/10.1182/blood-2018-99-110486
   Costa, L. J., Xing-Huang, J., & Hari, P. N. (2015). Disparities in utilization of autologous hematopoietic cell transplantation for treatment of multiple myeloma. *Biology of Blood and Marrow Transplant, 21*, 701–706.
   Fiala Joseph, M. A., Finney, D., Stockerl-Goldstein, K. E., Tomasson, M. H., DiPersio, D. F., Vij, R., & Wildes, T. M. (2015). Re: Disparities in utilization of autologous hematopoietic cell transplantation for treatment of multiple myeloma. *Biology of Blood and Marrow Transplantation, 21*, 1153–1154.
7. Eggers, P. W. (1995). Racial differences in access to kidney transplantation. *Health Care Financial Review, 17*(2), 89–103.
   Gaylin, D. S., Held, P. J., Port, F. K., et al. (1993). The impact of comorbid and sociodemographic factors on access to renal transplantation. *Journal of the American Medical Association, 269*(5), 603–608.
8. Eggers, P. W. (1995). Racial differences in access to kidney transplantation. *Health Care Financial Review, 17*(2), 89–103.
9. Purnell, T. S., Xu, P., Leca, N., & Hall, Y. N. (2013). Racial differences in determinants of live donor kidney transplantation in the United States. *American Journal of Transplantation, 13*, 1557–1565.
10. Donate Life American. https://www.donatelife.net/race-ethnicity-and-donation/
11. Patzera, R. E., Perrymana, J. P., Schragerc, J. D., Pastana, S., Amarale, D. S., Gazmararian, J. A., Klein, B. M., Kutnerfand, B. N., & McClellan, W. M. (2011). The role of race and poverty on steps to kidney transplantation in the southeastern United States. *American Journal of Transplantation, 12*, 358–368.
   Hall, Y. N., Choi, A. I., Xu, P., O'Hare, A. M., & Chertow, G. M. (2011). Racial ethnic differences in rates and determinants of deceased donor kidney transplantation. *Journal of the American Society of Nephrology, 22*, 743–751.
   Patzer, R. E., Amaral, S., Wasse, H., Volkova, N., Kleinbaum, D., & McClellan, W. M. (2009). Neighborhood poverty and racial disparities in kidney transplant waitlisting. *Journal of American Society of Nephrology, 20*, 1333–1340.
12. Held, P. J., Pauly, M. V., & Bovbjer, R. R. (1988). Access to kidney transplantation. Has the United States eliminated income and racial differences? *Archives of Intern Medicine, 148*(12), 2594–2600. https://doi.org/10.1001/archinte.148.12.2594
13. Malek, S. K., Keys, B. J., Kumar, S., Milford, E., & Tullius, S. G. (2010). Racial and ethnic disparities in kidney transplantation. *Transplant International, 24*(5), 419–424. https://doi.org/10.1111/j.1432-2277.2010.01205.x

14. Ayanian, J. Z., Cleary, P. D., Weissman, J. S., & Epstein, A. M. (1999). The effect of patient preferences on racial differences in access to renal transplantation. *The New England Journal of Medicine*, *341*, 1661–1669.
15. Fan, P. Y., Ashby, V. B., Fuller, D. S., et al. (2010). Access and outcomes among minority transplant patients, 1999-2008, with a focus on determinants of kidney graft survival. *American Journal of Transplantation*, *10*, 1090–1107. https://onlinelibrary.wiley.com/doi/epdf/10.1111/j.1600-6143.2009.03009.x
16. Johnson, J. D., Wicks, M. N., Milstead, J., Hartwig, M., & Hathaway, D. K. (2007). Racial and gender differences in quality of life following kidney transplantation. *The Journal of Nursing Scholarship*, *30*, 125–130.
17. Kaufman, S. R. (2013). Fairness and the tyranny of potential in kidney transplantation. *Current Anthropology*, *54*, 556–566, pp. 553.
18. Mazaris, E., & Papalois, V. E. (2008). Ethical issues in living donor kidney transplantation. *Experimental & Clinical Transplantation*, *4*(2), 485–497.

O'Hara Jr., J. F., Bramstedt, K., Flechner S., & Goldfarb, D. (2007). Ethical issues surrounding high-risk kidney recipients: Implications for the living donor. *Progress in Transplantation*, *17*(3), 180–182.

19. Bevans, M. F., Mitchell, S. A., & Marden, S. (2008). The symptom experience in the first 100 days following allogeneic hematopoietic stem cell transplantation (HSCT). *Supportive Care in Cancer*, *16*, 1243–1254.
20. Herrmann, S. M. S., et al. (2011). Long-term outcomes of patients with light chain amyloidosis (AL) after renal transplantation with or without stem cell transplantation. *Nephrology Dialysis Transplantation*, *26*(6), 2032–2036. https://doi.org/10.1093/ndt/gfr067
21. Pasternack, A., Ahonen, J., & Kuhlbäck, B. (1986). Renal transplantation in 45 patients with amyloidosis. *Transplantation*, *42*(6), 598–601. https://doi.org/10.1097/00007890-198612000-00005

INDEX

Milton Keynes UK
Ingram Content Group UK Ltd.
UKHW022058120524
442498UK00003B/29

9 781839 987670